On-Line Hemodiafiltration: The Journey and the Vision

Contributions to Nephrology

Vol. 175

Series Editor

Claudio Ronco Vicenza

On-Line Hemodiafiltration: The Journey and the Vision

Volume Editors

Gerd Krick Bad Homburg
Claudio Ronco Vicenza

42 figures, 19 in color, and 9 tables, 2011

KARGER Basel · Freiburg · Paris · London · New York · New Delhi · Bangkok · Beijing · Tokyo · Kuala Lumpur · Singapore · Sydney

Contributions to Nephrology
(Founded 1975 by Geoffrey M. Berlyne)

Gerd Krick
Fresenius SE & Co. KGaA
Else-Kröner-Straße 1
61352 Bad Homburg
Germany

Claudio Ronco
Department of Nephrology, Dialysis & Transplantation
International Renal Research Institute Vicenza
S. Bortolo Hospital, Viale Rodolfi, 37
36100 Vicenza, Italy

Library of Congress Cataloging-in-Publication Data

On-line hemodiafiltration : the journey and the vision / volume editors, Claudio Ronco, G. Krick.
p. ; cm. -- (Contributions to nephrology, ISSN 0302-5144 ; v. 175)
Includes bibliographical references and indexes.
ISBN 978-3-8055-9906-1 (hard cover : alk. paper) -- ISBN 978-3-8055-9907-8 (e-ISBN)
I. Ronco, C. (Claudio), 1951- II. Krick, Gerd. III. Series: Contributions to nephrology ; v. 175. 0302-5144
[DNLM: 1. Hemodiafiltration--instrumentation. 2. Hemodiafiltration--history. 3. Hemodiafiltration--methods. 4. History, 20th Century. 5. History, 21st Century. WJ 378]

617.4'61059--dc23

2011043129

Bibliographic Indices. This publication is listed in bibliographic services, including Current Contents® and Index Medicus.

Disclaimer. The statements, opinions and data contained in this publication are solely those of the individual authors and contributors and not of the publisher and the editor(s). The appearance of advertisements in the book is not a warranty, endorsement, or approval of the products or services advertised or of their effectiveness, quality or safety. The publisher and the editor(s) disclaim responsibility for any injury to persons or property resulting from any ideas, methods, instructions or products referred to in the content or advertisements.

Drug Dosage. The authors and the publisher have exerted every effort to ensure that drug selection and dosage set forth in this text are in accord with current recommendations and practice at the time of publication. However, in view of ongoing research, changes in government regulations, and the constant flow of information relating to drug therapy and drug reactions, the reader is urged to check the package insert for each drug for any change in indications and dosage and for added warnings and precautions. This is particularly important when the recommended agent is a new and/or infrequently employed drug.

www.karger.com
Printed in Germany on acid-free and non-aging paper (ISO 9706) by Bosch Druck, Ergolding
ISSN 0302–5144
e-ISSN 1662–2782
ISBN 978–3–8055–9906–1
e-ISBN 978–3–8055–9907–8

Contents

The Clinical Appraisal of On-Line Hemodiafiltration

Foreword

On-line hemodiafiltration represents a major technical development in the delivery of hemodialysis therapy. This modality combines the properties of increased diffusion available in current high-flux membranes with convective removal of between 6 and 30 liters per treatment. On-line hemodiafiltration requires the use of ultrapure water and online filtration of replacement fluid. This represents a major technical advance incorporated in FMC technology. This therapy has been successfully introduced in Europe and Asia and is routinely prescribed for dialysis patients in these regions.

The Fresenius Medical Care 5008 hemodialysis machine is used in the majority of on-line HDF treatments for use of HDF in Europe and other continents.

Dr. Emanuele Gatti, Management Board Member responsible for the 5008 HD machine development, made major contributions – both technically and managerially – to drive the development of the 5008 hemodialysis machine and on-line HDF.

This volume of *Contributions to Nephrology* describes the status of many online HDF clinical studies and the other major advances of dialysis patient care achieved during Emanuele's first 30 years in dialysis.

Emanuele and I have worked together for the past 25 years and I would like to congratulate him on his many accomplishments.

Ben Lipps, Boston

Preface

On-line HDF has gained today a high degree of popularity. The evolution of online HDF has been slow and gradual thanks to the contribution of many individuals. In Fresenius Medical Care, the tenacious activity of Dr. Gatti has guided the Company to overcome several hurdles. Development of new concepts of machine and dialyzer technologies have been the focus of several years of courageous investments, and different skills were needed to convince regulatory agencies about feasibility and safety. This book is in celebration for the 30th anniversary of Dr. Gatti's commitment to Fresenius Medical Care and a testimony of the story of success for the whole Company and for those who had the luck to share this experience in the past, present and future.

The book is divided in four parts: the first reports the technological development in both machine and fiber/dialyzer. The second represents the subsequent challenges encountered in the evolution of on-line HDF: from a host of several unmet clinical needs reported by the bedside operators (physicians and nurses) the Company has received the stimulus to identify and resolve the relevant technical issues responding to the specific needs with new products and innovative solutions. This part collects the testimony of clinical key opinion leaders who had been involved in the application of on-line HDF and had been instrumental in the evolution of some specific aspects of on-line HDF. The third is a comprehensive review of the clinical results achieved with on-line HDF since the inception of this technique to the present times in which it represents the clinical golden standard. This part includes the description of the process of adoption of on-line HDF as standard therapy in Fresenius Medical Care's own network of dialysis centers. The fourth and final part is dedicated to on-line HDF as a 'vision' for the future. New challenges and new ideas will be presented to document the never ending journey of research and development dedicated to kidney patients.

The book should hopefully fill a gap: it should teach how the vision in the future and the daily hard work together with a clear focus make the essential chemistry for success. The reader may benefit from contributions by different individuals who accompanied Dr. Gatti on the long journey. Dr. Gatti's vision was from the beginning based on listening to the attending physicians. Many instances of practices exist in medicines that do not/cannot await for clinical trials but are increasingly introduced with the common acceptance for a seeable patient benefit. Only years after this vision came the demonstration of a significant benefit in survival of patients on on-line HDF. This would have been possible, if, even in the absence of such a recognition, the technology would have not made this modality of current use and the regulatory issues solved.

Claudio Ronco, Vicenza

Homage

Hemodiafiltration, developed from the combination of hemodialysis and hemofiltration, is considered to be the most effective current procedure to remove uremic toxins from the blood of kidney patients. Historically, the clinical use of hemodiafiltration was for many years limited due to the cost burden related to the large amount of sterile replacement fluid needed. The solution offered was an on-line preparation of replacement fluid from standard dialysate by means of membrane filtration. Industry opened to this concept quite early and worked on various technical solutions between the early 80ies and the late 90ies before real state-of-the-art systems became commercially available on a broad basis. This volume of *Contributions to Nephrology* reviews in particular the activities of initially Fresenius and later Fresenius Medical Care in this field and identifies major concepts and prototypes up to today's commercially available high-end product – the 5008 therapy system – where on-line HDF finally became integrated as a standard component.

Over the years, as a member or Chairman of the Boards of Fresenius and Fresenius Medical Care, I have initiated and encouraged the development of the scientific, medical and technical basis for a commercial on-line hemodiafiltration system. This development, and that of the accompanying innovative 5008 therapy system, was driven by the significant technical and managerial contributions of Dr. Emanuele Gatti of the Fresenius Medical Care Management Board. Through his tremendous dedication, he succeeded in overcoming multifarious hurdles to reach today's acceptance of on-line hemodiafiltration as a new standard in renal replacement therapy. His technical, managerial and business experience were unremittingly devoted to convincing the medical community and regulatory authorities of this vision of the future.

This book summarizes different aspects of this historical development pathway as experienced by those who have worked close to him for many years and who have shared his commitment to on-line hemodiafiltration.

Gerd Krick, Bad Homburg

Krick G, Ronco C (eds): On-Line Hemodiafiltration: The Journey and the Vision.
Contrib Nephrol. Basel, Karger, 2011, vol 175, pp 1–14

Historical Milestones of a Long Pathway

Thomas Roy

Fresenius Medical Care Deutschland GmbH, R&D International, Bad Homburg, Germany

Abstract

Hemodiafiltration (HDF), developed from the combination of hemodialysis and hemofiltration, is considered to be the most effective current procedure to remove uremic toxins from the blood of kidney patients. Historically, the clinical use of HDF was for many years limited due to the cost burden related to the large amount of sterile volume replacement fluid needed. The solution offered was on-line preparation of replacement fluid from standard dialysate by means of membrane filtration. Industry opened to this concept quite early and worked on various technical solutions between the early 1980s and the late 1990s before real state-of-the-art systems became commercially available on a broad basis. This article reviews in particular the activities of initially Fresenius and later Fresenius Medical Care in this field and identifies major concepts and prototypes up to today's commercially available high-end product – the 5008 therapy system – where on-line HDF finally became integrated as a standard component.

From 'Ultrafiltration' to 'Diafiltration' and 'Hemofiltration'

To review the historical pathway from the early days to modern on-line hemodiafiltration (HDF) necessarily requires starting with hemofiltration (HF) as developed and carefully introduced into clinical practice during the late 1960s/early 1970s. To the author's knowledge and as referenced by other sources, the first paper reporting preclinical trials to correct the uremic conditions of dogs by means of 'ultrafiltration' dates from 1947. There, Mailonov and Korzon [1] describe an 'ultrafiltration' procedure in normal and nephrectomized dogs where the gained ultrafiltrate volume was manually replaced by a standard Ringer-lactate solution. Due to the high hydraulic resistance of the used tubular cellophane membrane assemblies, the achieved filtrate volume was so discouraging low (50–70 ml/h at effective pressures between 760 and 900 mm Hg) that the authors concluded that the '. . .procedure with the apparatus employed (is) unsuitable for man. . .' and clearly favored the Kolff drum dialyzer approach.

Retrospectively, it seems fair to say that the lack of membrane materials with low hydraulic resistances over the following two decades prevented repetition and expansion of these early experiments. A paper by Henderson et al. [2] from 1967 on the in vitro evaluation of the newly developed Amicon Diaflo membrane is considered to mark the resumption of ultrafiltration for extracorporeal detoxification purposes. The process used for removing toxins from blood by convective transport in this paper was termed 'diafiltration', which caused some confusion in later years before the name was finally converted to 'hemofiltration' by Dr. Benjamin Burton from the NIH during the historic Braunlage Conference in 1976 [see 3].

The transfer of the rediscovered HF procedure to clinical routine proceeded with extreme caution during the following years, moving in several steps from animal experiments to humans and by scaling up the amount of required fluid exchange. An impressive description of this really pioneering work and the inherent risks and uncertainties was given retrospectively by Henderson [4] himself in 2003. In fairness, it must be acknowledged here that the first reliable clinical data for patients on long-term maintenance HF were generated by German researchers such as Quellhorst and others in the years after 1971.

Due to the early interest of German nephrologists in HF, it was not by chance that some of the first commercially available systems for HF were developed by German companies such as Sartorius/Göttingen and Dialysetechnik/Karlsruhe [5]. This clinical and technical progress in Europe was certainly influenced by the availability of membranes with high hydraulic permeabilities, such as the famous AN69 [6, 7] or the disc filters by Sartorius [see 8]. It should be mentioned that, unlike early hemodialysis (HD), HF was supported from the very beginning by thorough theoretical analyses regarding solute transport, and this finally led to a very straightforward approach in terms of clinical application [9, 10].

HF, however, was burdened from the start by two different factors: financially, by the high cost for large amounts of intravenous replacement fluids, and medically, compared to HD, by the lower efficacy of the procedure in terms of low molecular weight clearances [e.g. 11]). Compensation for the HF-related increase in systemic urea concentration required larger amounts of substitution fluid (given in predilution mode to increase convective fluxes) and further exacerbated the cost aspect of maintenance HF. The author remembers that it needed some courage and 'acclimatization' in the first maintenance HF patients in the light of their otherwise improved status to simply tolerate these

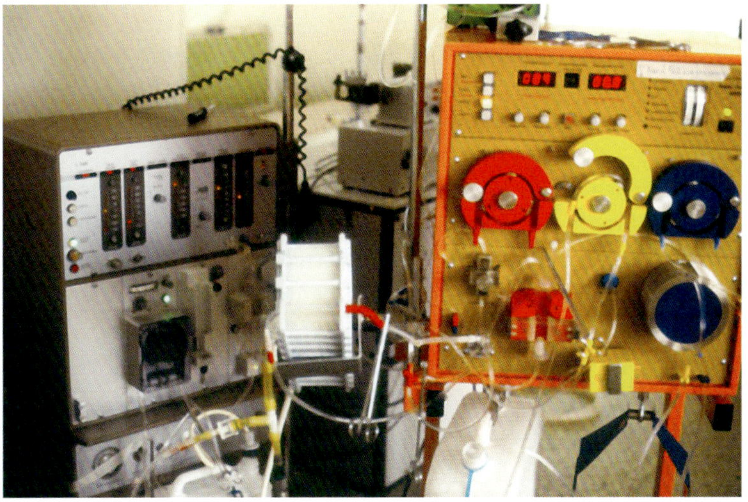

Fig. 1. Fresenius A2008C (left) and Sartorius Haemoprocessor (right) in Giessen (Germany) simultaneously performing HD and HF via a shared RP-6 high-flux dialyzer. Courtesy of Prof. Volker Wizemann, Giessen.

elevated urea levels for the sake of reasonable expenditure for substitution fluid.

Hemodiafiltration as the Ultimate Modality

It seems to be impossible to retrospectively determine the source of the idea of combining HD and HF in a single procedure. Definitely the working group of Prof. Leber from the University Hospital Giessen/Germany in 1976 [12] started with a procedure where HD and HF were performed within one single RP-6 filter in order to maximize solute removal over the whole sieving range of the filter. The paper reporting these experiments was published in 1978 and is commonly considered to be the birth certificate of HDF [13]. Therein, the authors describe a procedure where fluid removal by ultrafiltration and fluid reinfusion from an intravenous fluid reservoir was performed by means of manual control of the respective pumps under the guidance of the patient's bed scale in order to achieve the desired fluid balance. The HD circuit of the treatment was operated in parallel by a standard Drake Willock HD machine. This cumbersome way of performing HDF was improved in later years by using the volumetric fluid-balancing feature of a Fresenius A2008C HD system in conjunction with a gravimetric fluid-balancing system to control the convective flux conditions in an automated way [14]. Fortunately, a remarkable photograph of one of these early HDF set-ups is available from Giessen (see fig. 1).

Fresenius and Hemodiafiltration

The Fresenius R&D archive documents that some of the company's interest in the mid-1970s was focused on equipment for HF while, in parallel, a new-generation HD system – the later A2008 – was under development. Since the HD project began earlier and certainly was the more challenging one (not less challenging than the development of the first single-pass HD machine with volumetric UF control in an autoclavable stainless steel version), the company's HF activities never led to anything more than a combination of various components for performing HF in a manually controlled way. However, other companies developed dedicated HF equipment at this time (Sartorius/Göttingen, Dialysetechnik/Karlsruhe or Gambro/Lund).

Due to contacts with the Giessen group of Leber and Wizemann, we became aware of their very successful and convincing developments regarding HDF and saw the possibility of combining the meanwhile ready A2008 dialysis machine with a Sartorius Haemoprocessor. In a resulting cooperation between Fresenius and Sartorius, the first commercially available system for HDF, the so-called ABG-1, was developed and introduced to the market. As described in figure 2, the closed hydraulic circuit of the A2008 provided a perfect platform for extension towards HDF, a feature from which even today's Fresenius HD machines still benefit. The final device (shown in figure 3) was a slightly modified A2008 equipped with a substitution fluid heater and pump, and with the Sartorius-manufactured ABG (i.e. the German abbreviation for automatic balancing device) on top. The ABG was produced in two different versions (the later ABG-II without cooperation with Sartorius) for all Fresenius 2008 series HD machines.

All Fresenius activities regarding HDF benefited from a strong and enduring support from the top level management. This was first provided by the person of Gerd Krick and later by Emanuele Gatti. Gerd Krick, then the board member responsible for the Medical Devices Division, clearly recognized the potential of the new treatment modality and the advantageous technical position of Fresenius in this context. This position was further improved by the upcoming polysulfone high-flux dialyzer, the well-known Fresenius F-60, which became the yardstick for synthetic, high-performance, biocompatible dialyzers for many years.

The Need to Go 'On-Line'

As promising as the clinical results of the newly introduced technique were its expansion into the field of treating maintenance dialysis patients clearly remained below expectations and below the potential of the method. In Europe, typical HDF countries were France, Germany and Italy, but even in these

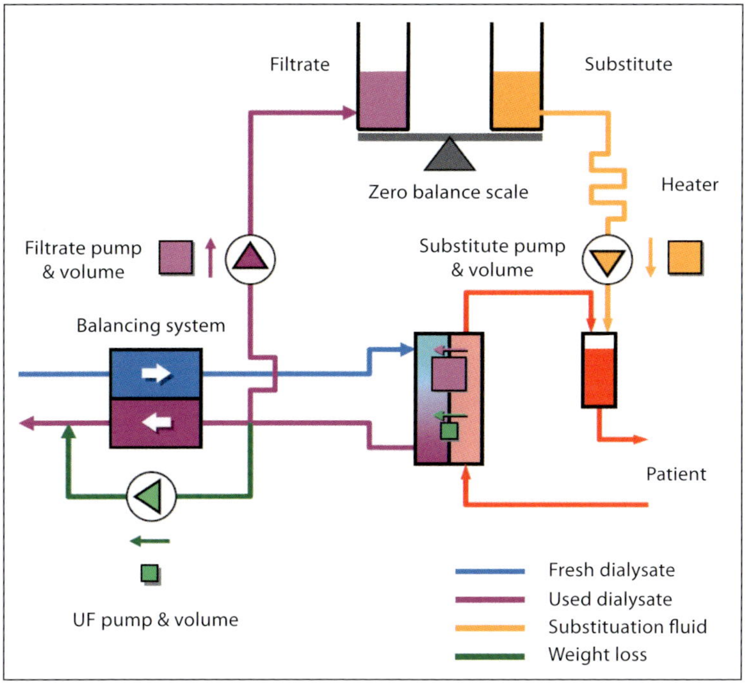

Fig. 2. This schematic diagram shows why the hydraulic circuit of an A2008 machine was ideal for retrofitting with a HDF module: an added filtrate pump removed fluid from the spent dialysate stream. Due to the closed hydraulic system of the A2008, exactly this amount of fluid was removed from the patient (compare squares indicating volumes). Under control of a zero balance scale, an equal amount of substitution fluid was given back to the patient. The desired weight loss was achieved with the machine's standard UF pump.

countries HDF was not common practice and remained fairly isolated in the hands of some convinced and enthusiastic medical doctors. Among the different reasons for the hesitant application of HDF, financial constraints always played a major role due to the required large volumes of intravenous grade electrolyte solution.

However, a solution (again by Henderson et al.) for the financial dilemma appeared in 1978 when they successfully produced large amounts of intravenous grade electrolyte solution from standard dialysate by cold filtration in a batch-like mode [15] and in a true 'on-line' mode [16] through Amicon XP-50 filters. In batch mode, filter integrity was demonstrated by means of blue dextran challenging (MW 2×10^6 daltons) and 'classic' tests of the product fluid (culturing, LAL). In on-line mode, pretreatment integrity testing using blue dextran was combined with sufficient filter redundancy (two filters). This filter redundancy strategy is still in use in today's state-of-the-art on-line systems.

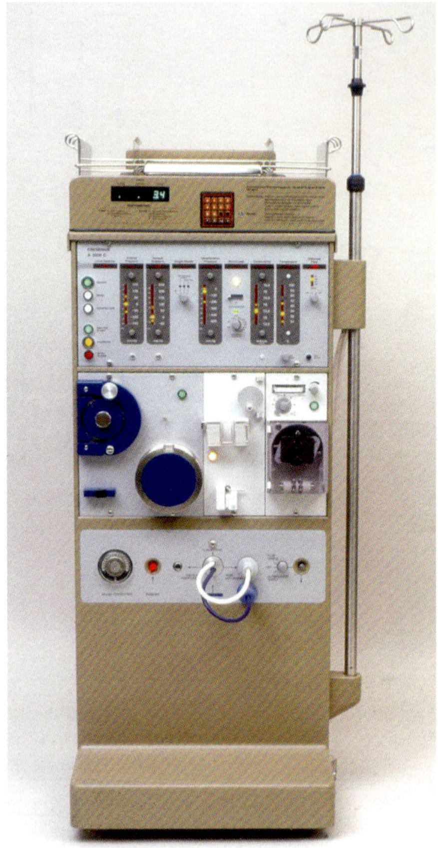

Fig. 3. The first commercially available system for HDF: a Fresenius A2008C with the ABG-1 Hemodiafiltration Module, a joint development of Fresenius AG (Bad Homburg, Germany) and Sartorius AG (Göttingen, Germany). Source: FMC R&D archive.

Thus, Henderson's ASAIO paper [16] can be considered the birth document of modern on-line HF/HDF technology. This is somewhat ironical in medical devices history considering the fact that for regulatory reasons this type of technology in the USA is virtually still unused.

Which Membranes for On-Line Filters?

Interest in on-line substitution fluid preparation fortunately developed in parallel to the introduction of new synthetic capillary filter membranes such as polysulfone (PSu) and polyamide (PA). Filters with these new membranes were high-flux types with corresponding high clearances and low hydraulic resistances. The high water permeability of these membranes, combined with the standard pressures and pressure drops in an extracorporeal circuit containing a dialyzer, caused a new phenomenon called 'backfiltration' [see 17]. This term describes a situation where, due to local pressure gradients from the dialysate compartment towards the blood compartment of the filter, fluid from the dialysate side enters the patient's blood. This potential hazard prompted a careful investigation of these membranes regarding rejection and adsorption of various microbiological contaminants normally present in standard dialysate. Although there was early evidence that especially asymmetric synthetic polymers, such as PSu and PA, provided excellent barriers against the relevant microbiological burdens [see e.g. 18] the concern regarding the safety of high-flux membranes was kept alive by various corporate marketing departments for many years. However, medical science and industry quickly recognized the potential of these new membranes not only as a safe barrier against microbiological dialysate contamination but – even more important – to serve as suitable dialysate filters and to allow the desired production of intravenous grade fluid from standard dialysate. It was certainly not by chance that the industrial corporations focusing on PSu (Fresenius AG, Bad Homburg, Germany) and PA (Gambro AB, Lund, Sweden) were the pioneers and the drivers when it came to equipment for HF/HDF with on-line preparation of substitution fluid.

Fresenius and On-Line Fluid Preparation

The meanwhile available A2008C HD machine with its volumetric fluid-balancing systems offered a perfect platform for integration of not only a HF/HDF procedure but also the feature of on-line fluid preparation. The respective activities inside Fresenius were primarily driven by Gerd Krick, at that time CEO of the Medical Devices Division, and Hans Dietrich Polaschegg, the Director for R&D Medical Devices. Figure 4 shows the facsimile of a 1986 order from Gerd Krick to enforce and finish the development and the market introduction of a system for on-line HDF. The letter perfectly describes the far-sighted attitude and future intention of Fresenius as started by Gerd Krick and continued by Emanuele Gatti until today.

However, the early prototypes of on-line HDF systems were far from being elegant and user-friendly as they included a lot of time-consuming and essential manual handling steps. Figure 5 – without further details being discussed here – shows the flow path of a 1984 system which was clinically tested in Giessen, Germany. Apart from all the manual elements in this system, it already represents the configuration Fresenius followed from the beginning until today: volume control is provided by the balancing system of the HD machine, and fluid preparation is done by means of two redundant large-surface-area, multiple-use PSu filters. For safety reasons, this configuration requires a predialysis functional test for filter integrity [19]. This follows from the adopted concept of two redundant filters as a safeguard against a first fault as required by the various safety standards for medical devices. For a detailed analysis of the safety concept

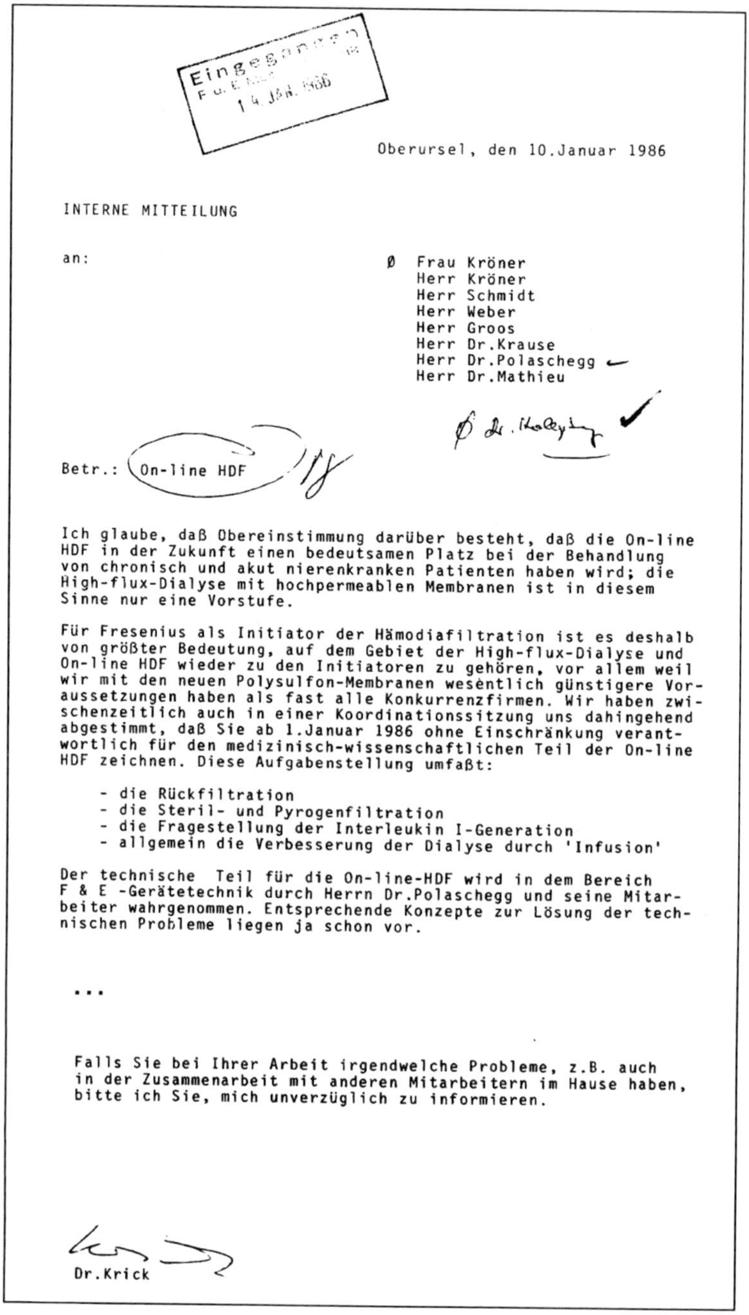

Eingegangen F. u. E. 14. JAN. 1986

Oberursel, den 10.Januar 1986

INTERNE MITTEILUNG

an:

Ø Frau Kröner
Herr Kröner
Herr Schmidt
Herr Weber
Herr Groos
Herr Dr.Krause
Herr Dr.Polaschegg
Herr Dr.Mathieu

Betr.: On-line HDF

Ich glaube, daß Übereinstimmung darüber besteht, daß die On-line HDF in der Zukunft einen bedeutsamen Platz bei der Behandlung von chronisch und akut nierenkranken Patienten haben wird; die High-flux-Dialyse mit hochpermeablen Membranen ist in diesem Sinne nur eine Vorstufe.

Für Fresenius als Initiator der Hämodiafiltration ist es deshalb von größter Bedeutung, auf dem Gebiet der High-flux-Dialyse und On-line HDF wieder zu den Initiatoren zu gehören, vor allem weil wir mit den neuen Polysulfon-Membranen wesentlich günstigere Voraussetzungen haben als fast alle Konkurrenzfirmen. Wir haben zwischenzeitlich auch in einer Koordinationssitzung uns dahingehend abgestimmt, daß Sie ab 1.Januar 1986 ohne Einschränkung verantwortlich für den medizinisch-wissenschaftlichen Teil der On-line HDF zeichnen. Diese Aufgabenstellung umfaßt:

- die Rückfiltration
- die Steril- und Pyrogenfiltration
- die Fragestellung der Interleukin I-Generation
- allgemein die Verbesserung der Dialyse durch 'Infusion'

Der technische Teil für die On-line-HDF wird in dem Bereich F & E -Gerätetechnik durch Herrn Dr.Polaschegg und seine Mitarbeiter wahrgenommen. Entsprechende Konzepte zur Lösung der technischen Probleme liegen ja schon vor.

...

Falls Sie bei Ihrer Arbeit irgendwelche Probleme, z.B. auch in der Zusammenarbeit mit anderen Mitarbeitern im Hause haben, bitte ich Sie, mich unverzüglich zu informieren.

Dr.Krick

Fig. 4. Written order and rationale by Fresenius AG Board Member Dr. G. Krick to boost and finish development of the scientific, medical and technical basis for a commercial on-line HDF system. Source: FMC R&D archive, permission G. Krick (author's translation): *'. . .I believe there is agreement that on-line HDF in future will play an important role in the treatment of acute or chronic kidney patients; in this sense high-flux dialysis with highly permeable*

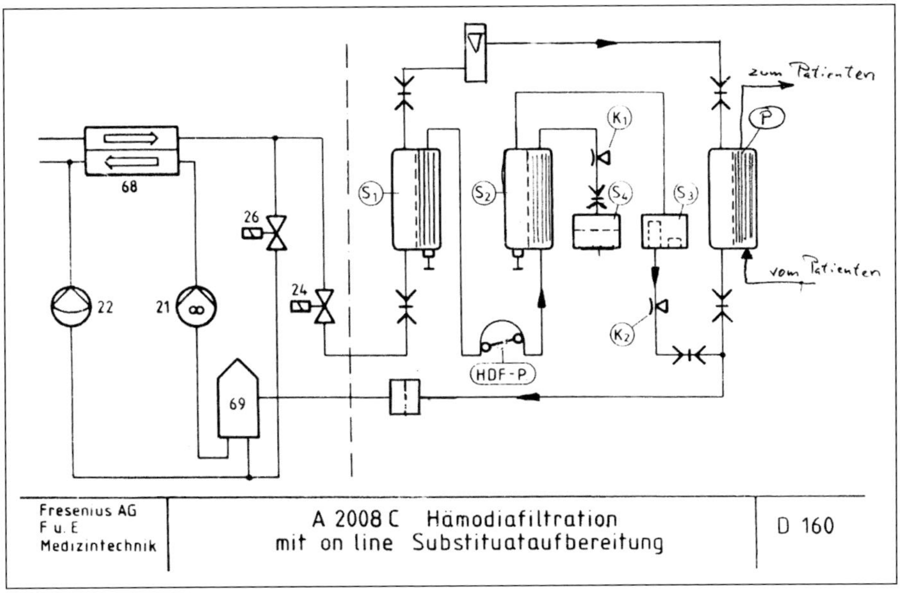

Fig. 5. Experimental on-line HDF system for the A2008C HD machine from 1984, including redundant fluid filters, various additional filters and clamps for manual filter integrity testing. Source: FMC R&D archive.

for HDF systems comprising on-line fluid preparation, see Polaschegg and Roy [20].

Apart from the need for dialysate ultrafilters as major elements for on-line HDF, we were always convinced about the benefit of having ultrafiltered dialysate in every standard HD treatment. Consequently, early R&D activities, in parallel to the development of on-line systems, led to the introduction of special dialysate filters. These filters (later known under the brand name 'Diasafe®') were optimized in several steps for their intended use together with Fresenius HD machines. The process included membrane adaptation, fiber potting, resistance to damage during chemical and thermal procedures, connection

membranes is just a preliminary stage. For Fresenius as initiator of hemodiafiltration it is of outermost importance to belong to the pioneers of high-flux dialysis and on-line HDF again, especially because we have a much better position compared to nearly all competitors due to the new polysulfone membrane. . . . We meanwhile agreed that – effective January 1st, 1986 and without any constraints – you will be responsible for the medical and scientific concept of on-line HDF. This task includes (a) backfiltration, (b) sterile and pyrogen filtration, (c) the question of IL-1 generation, (d) the general improvement of dialysis by means of 'infusion'. The technical part of on-line HDF is addressed already in R&D Medical Devices by Dr. Polaschegg and his co-workers. Concepts to solve the technical problems already are available. . . . In case you face any problems during your work, including problems regarding cooperation with in-house employees, you are asked to inform me immediately. . .'

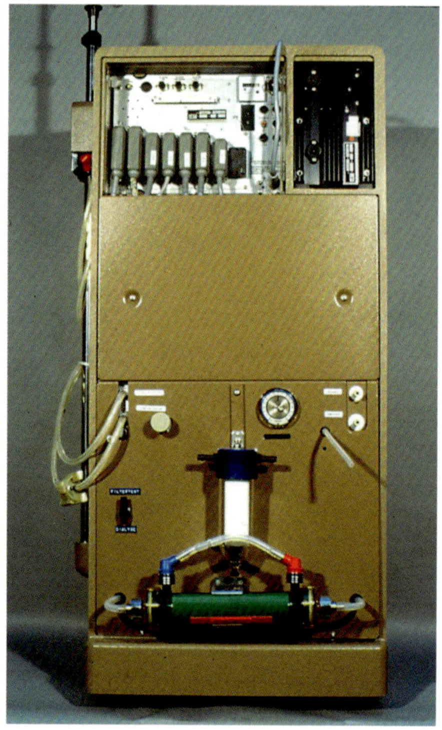

Fig. 6. The A2008C HD machine with early Diasafe® dialysate ultrafilter installation (1986). Source: FMC R&D archive.

technology and, most importantly, a sufficiently sensitive and finally automated filter integrity test. Figure 6 shows an early A2008C machine from 1986 with one of these specially adapted filters.

The first approved and commercially available on-line HDF system by Fresenius (fig. 7) was ready in 1987, when it was approved by the German TÜV according to the Medical Devices Act ('Medizingeräteverordnung' MedGV) in its 1985 version. This particular approval procedure was a new challenge for the manufacturer as well as for the test house since the existing relevant standards (VDE DIN 0750 part 1/05.1982 and VDE DIN 0750 part 206/09.1984) did not contain any explicit statements about procedures or safety measures for the on-line preparation of intravenous infusion fluid. A positive result, however, could be achieved by an appropriate interpretation of existing standards in the light of their general intention to provide first fault safety as required for this type of equipment.

The A2008 on-line HDF system comprised two special filters, a dialysate filter and a so-called HDF filter. The HDF filter could be vented via a GoreTex membrane to allow the required initial filter integrity test. The test procedure was partly automated although it had to be manually started and the results had to be checked and judged by the operator. In an improved version, which

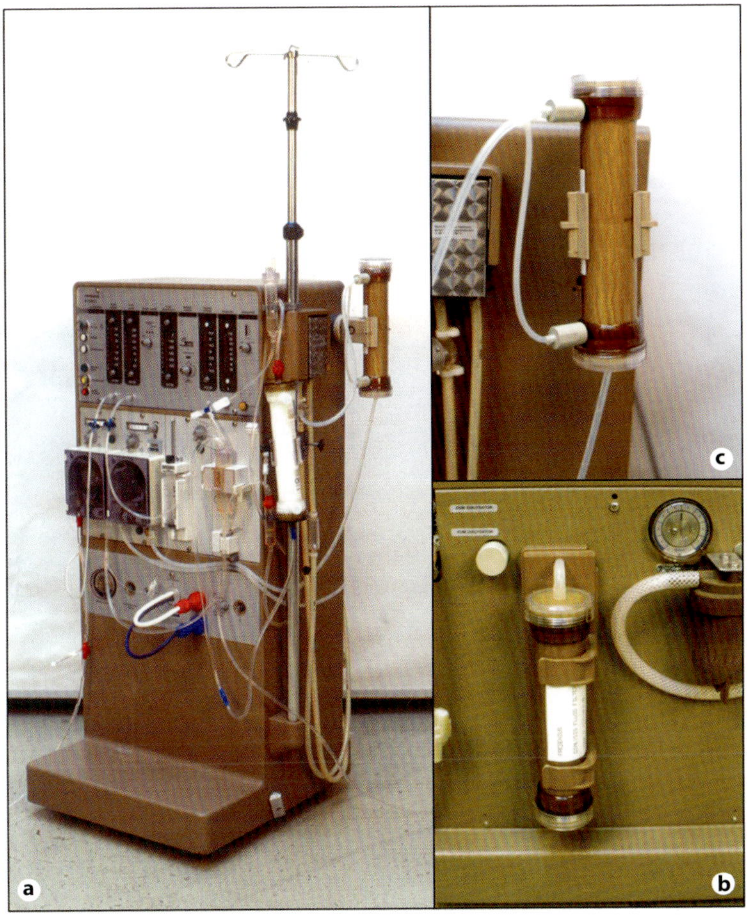

Fig. 7. First approved and commercially available Fresenius on-line HDF system for the HD machine A2008C/D/E (1987): (**a**) overall view, (**b**) Diasafe® dialysate ultrafilter, and (**c**) on-line HDF-filter. Source: FMC R&D archive.

included a fully automated filter integrity test, the system also was used in the FMC 4008 HD machine before it was replaced by the current Online plus™ system (see further down).

Retrospectively, one has to admit that these early systems still were quite cumbersome and had a high potential for further improvement and automation. Nevertheless, they opened the way towards a cost-efficient, high-performance renal replacement therapy. Sales figures, mostly on the basis of individual prescriptions by a physician for a particular patient, remained low and the systems stayed in the hands of few interested nephrologists. However, looking back, one must say that this period of subdued and limited use provided the required basis for gathering data and experiences with this new kind of technology.

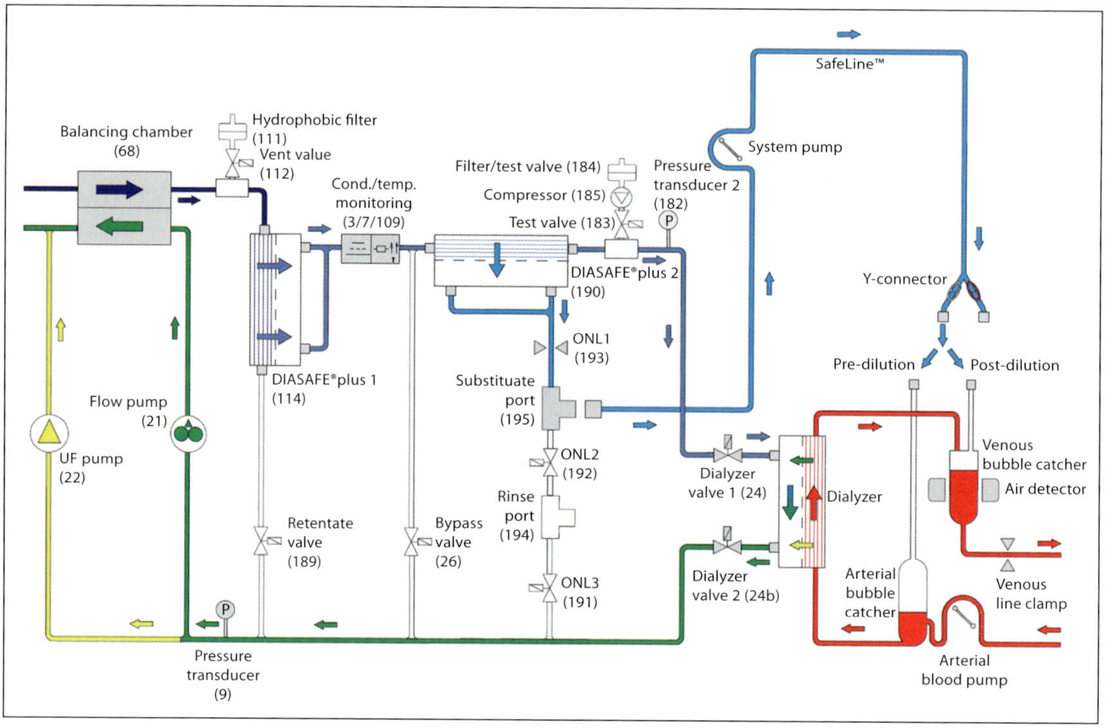

Fig. 8. Flow path for the Fresenius Online plus® hemodiafiltration system. Source: FMC product documentation.

Our Standard in On-Line HDF: Online plus™

In 1998, after summarizing all the experiences collected over more than 10 years with a newly designed system, Fresenius introduced the basis of the current technology under the brand name 'Online plus™'. The required approval procedure for on-line fluid preparation systems at that time had been clarified on the basis of the so-called 'Medical Devices Directive' [21] and a detailed interpretation given by Pirovano [22] in 1998. These virtually cleared the last hurdles for broad clinical use of on-line HDF in Europe.

Apart from fully automated procedures implemented in the Online plus™ system at the machine side (filter testing, monitoring of proper connections, etc.), a new filter generation under the name 'Diasafe® plus' came on the market. While earlier filters had a certain heritage from standard dialyzer technology, the Diasafe® plus, a 2.2-m² PSu filter, comprised special, new technologies (potting, connector design, etc.) to ensure handling comfort, excellent hygiene and maximum filter lifetime. The hydraulic flow path of the system is shown in figure 8. The new arrangement of the two Diasafe® plus filters in dead-end (filter 1) and in cross-flow mode (filter 2) provides effective use of the freshly prepared dialysate and – in parallel – prevents potentially dangerous build-up of microbiological burdens at the retentate side of the filters [see 23] by cyclic rinse procedures performed at the inlet side of filter 1.

To achieve cost-effective operation of the system, both filters are designed for multiple use over a life period of 3 months or 100 treatments (whichever comes first); a third disposable filter element, as used in other systems [see 20], is not necessary. This set-up requires a functional pretreatment filter integrity test as is always used in Fresenius systems. This test, based on the unique hydraulic configuration of Fresenius HD machines and the properties of the PSu membranes used in the filters, could be further improved [24] and fully automated. The growing experience with the new technology even allowed the defined exposure of the filter membranes to an otherwise critical substance such as bleach – this was urgently required by the dialysis clinics for cleaning purposes [25]. Since on-line prepared fluid was proven to be safe, it was consequently also considered for application in other steps of the dialysis procedure, such as priming of the extracorporeal circuit, applying volume boli and return of blood at the end of the treatment. These features of modern on-line HDF/HF systems further improve the financial footprint of these highly effective treatment modalities.

Exciting New Technologies One Day Become Common Standards

In 2005, after nearly 20 years of research, development and gathering experience, it was decided that, rather that just being an option, on-line HDF would be a standard procedure of the newly introduced Fresenius HD machine.

On this historical path towards today's therapy systems, the Lister Renal Unit from Stevenage was (among others) a much appreciated partner over many years. The author remembers a conversation with Roger Greenwood about on-line HDF from that time, where one of Dr. Greenwood's answers was that HDF (and for financial reasons on-line HDF) would just '. . .be common sense. . .'.

Sometimes it is as simple as this.

References

1 Malinow MR, Korzon W: An experimental method for obtaining an ultrafiltrate of blood. J Lab Clin Med 1947;32:461–471.

2 Henderson LW, Besarab A, Michaels A, Bluemle LW: Blood purification by ultrafiltration and fluid replacement (diafiltration). Trans ASAI0 1967;13:216–226.

3 Quellhorst E: Geschichte der Hämofiltration. Nieren- und Hochdruckkrankheiten (in German), Jahrgang 38, Nr 2/2009, pp 43–47.

4 Henderson LW: The beginning of clinical hemofiltration: a personal account. ASAIO J 2003;49:513–517.

5 Kramer P, Wigger W, Matthaei D, Langescheid C, Rieger J, Fuchs C, Rumpf KW, Scheler F: Clinical experience with continuously monitored fluid balance in automatic hemofiltration. Artif Organs 1978;2:147–149.
6 Funck-Brentano JL, Sausse A, Vantelon J, Granger A, Zingraff J, Man NK: A new disposable plate-kidney. Trans Am Soc Artif Intern Organs 1969;15:127–130.
7 Man NK, Granger A, Rondon-Nucete M, Zingraff J, Jungers P, Sausse A, Funck-Brentano JL: One year follow-up of short dialysis with a membrane highly permeable to middle molecules. Proc Eur Dial Transplant Assoc 1973;10:236–246.
8 Nussbaumer D, Perl H: Einflussgrössen bei der Hämofiltration (in German). Wissenschaftliche Informationen Fresenius, Nephrologie, Heft 2/1078, 145–155.
9 Colton CK, Henderson LW, Ford CA, Lysaght MJ: Kinetics of hemodiafiltration. I. In vitro transport characteristics of a hollow-fiber blood ultrafilter. J Lab Clin Med 1975;85:355–371.
10 Henderson LW, Colton CK, Ford CA: Kinetics of hemodiafiltration. II. Clinical characterization of a new blood cleansing modality. J Lab Clin Med 1975;85:372–391.
11 Baldamus CA, Schoeppe W, Koch KM: Comparison of haemodialysis and post-dilution haemofiltration on an unselected dialysis population. Proc Eur Dial Transplant Assoc 1978;15:228–235.
12 Wizemann V, Rawer P, Schmidt H, Techert F, Schuetterle G: Efficiency of hemodialysis, hemofiltration and hemodiafiltration; in Schuetterle G, Wizemann V, Seyffart G (eds): Hemodiafiltration. Proceedings 1. Symposion Giessen 1981. Oberursel/Ts, Verlag Hygieneplan, 1982.
13 Leber HW, Wizemann V, Goubeaud G, Rawer P, Schütterle G: Simultaneous hemofiltration/hemodialysis: an effective alternative to hemofiltration and conventional hemodialysis in the treatment of uremic patients. Clin Nephrol 1978;9:115–121.
14 Leber HW, Wizemann V, Techert F: Simultaneous hemofiltration/hemodialysis: short- and long-term tolerance. Introduction of a system for automatic fluid replacement. Artif Organs 1980;4:108–112.
15 Henderson LW, Beans E: Successful production of sterile pyrogen-free electrolyte solution by ultrafiltration. Kidney Int 1978;14:522–525.
16 Henderson LW, Sanfelippo ML, Beans E: 'On line' preparation of sterile pyrogen-free electrolyte solution. Trans Am Soc Artif Intern Organs 1978;24:465–467.
17 Stiller S, Mann H, Brunner H: Backfiltration in hemodialysis with highly permeable membranes. Contrib Nephrol. Basel, Karger, 1985, vol 46, pp 23–32.
18 Bommer J, Becker KP, Urbaschek R, Ritz E, Urbaschek B: No evidence for endotoxin transfer across high-flux polysulfone membranes. Clin Nephrol 1987;27:278–282.
19 Polaschegg HD, Mathieu B: EP 0189 561, priority 05.12.1985.
20 Polaschegg HD, Roy T: Technical aspects of online hemodiafiltration. Contrib Nephrol. Basel, Karger, 2007, vol 158, pp 68–79.
21 Community Directive 93/42/EEC on Medical Devices: Official Journal of the European Communities, No L169, 12 July 1993.
22 Pirovano D: Regulatory issues for on-line haemodiafiltration. Nephrol Dial Transplant 1998;13(suppl 5):21–39.
23 Nederlof B: European Patent EP 0692 268, priority 13.07.1994.
24 Wamsiedler R, Mathieu B: European Patent EP 0763 367, priority 16.09.1995.
25 Weber C, Groetsch W, Schlotter S, Mitteregger R, Falkenhagen D: Novel online infusate-assisted dialysis system performs microbiologically safely. Artif Organs 2000;24:323–328.

Dr. Thomas Roy
Fresenius Medical Care Deutschland GmbH
R&D International, Daimlerstrasse 15
DE–61352 Bad Homburg (Germany)
Tel. +49 6172 609 2397, E-Mail thomas.roy@fmc-ag.com

Krick G, Ronco C (eds): On-Line Hemodiafiltration: The Journey and the Vision.
Contrib Nephrol. Basel, Karger, 2011, vol 175, pp 15–26

Polysulfone: The Development of a Membrane for Convective Therapies

Klaus Heilmann · Torsten Keller

Fresenius Medical Care Deutschland GmbH, Membrane & Filter Development, St. Wendel, Germany

Abstract

The polysulfone membrane was developed as a membrane for convective dialysis therapies at the beginning of the 1980s. The target was to produce a higher-permeable membrane on the basis of synthetic polymers, such as polysulfone. The development of a membrane with high permeability went hand in hand with a technology development that finally presented as an essential precondition for the success of the polysulfone membrane. This article describes the development phase of the polysulfone membrane using to-date unpublished extracts of the project report of the polysulfone membrane and commenting these from today's perspective.

Convective renal replacement therapies such as on-line hemodiafiltration (HDF) place high demands on the membranes used – demands that could only be met through the lessons learned during the development of polysulfone membranes.

The history of development of the polysulfone membrane for HDF therapy began with a re-orientation regarding the basic membrane material that, at that time, was predominantly cellulose. The motivation for this new beginning was the need for membranes with a higher permeability in order to support convective hemodialysis processes, coupled with the need to prevent a drop in leukocyte numbers during treatment (leukopenia), neither of which were possible with cellulose membranes. Different synthetic membranes for different applications had already been on the market when first interest in using these synthetic membranes for hemodialysis arose at the end of the 1970s. Examples were polyacrylnitrile (Asahi), polyamide, PMMA (Teijin) and also even a polysulfone

(Amicon). These activities started in different companies that were interested in improving dialysis and that recognized the potential of these new membranes, albeit certainly unaware of all advantages of synthetic membranes at that point of time (e.g. Amicon, Asahi, Gambro, Sartorius). These advantages only developed in the course of use and finally accounted for the later predominance of synthetic membranes. In the beginning, existing knowledge of the production of polysulfone membranes was rudimentary, forming only the basis for the subsequent development of a polysulfone dialysis membrane. The first aim of this development was optimization of the membrane permeability and retention properties for hemodialysis, hemofiltration and HDF applications, together with achievement of good hemocompatibility, stability, high quality and low production costs – all of which together constituted preconditions for a competitive product. Although some predevelopment had already been done, fulfillment of these preconditions required enormous efforts in the field of both product and technology development. For example, it was not possible to buy the necessary process technology in a ready-to-use form; new technological developments were necessary to facilitate creation of an economically successful product with high quality and constant properties. Within this context it was necessary to develop numerous detailed solutions enabling the mass production of dialysis membranes. This allowed scale-up of production from the early experimental process of lab-scale production of polysulfone capillary membranes in very limited qualities. An as yet unpublished report on the development of the polysulfone dialysis membrane provides interesting insight into these times of change, problems that arose and, in many cases, solutions still valid today [K. Heilmann: Project In-House Production of Hollow Fibers, unpubl. data, 1983]:

'*1. Initial situation and planning target*

Already in 1979, the management board knew about the necessity to develop and produce membranes (hollow fibers) for the dialysis.

Because there was no in-house know-how available about membrane technology, a co-operation with the company Berghof was decided. At the beginning of 1980 a know-how and license agreement was concluded with Berghof.

The advantage of this agreement mainly consisted in the acquirement of basic knowledge, such as spinning recipe and dry-wet spinning technology, as well as in the time saving – the learning process would have taken at least 1 additional year.

The existing basic knowledge was planned to be supplemented by an in-house development in 1980 and a fiber production should be set up. The aim was the production of a capillary hemofilter.

The question for us in St. Wendel was whether to decide for the primitive but quick realization or for the long way leading to better results but probably too late.

In many project phases I decided for the long but better way (often on my own initiative, against resistance and using my complete leeway for decisions).

Emotionally I argue that the whole medical technology area of the company can only survive in case an in-house production of membranes will be successful. This emotion is now supported by the following facts:

- Cellulose membranes are more and more becoming the subject of gossip. We are practically committed to our suppliers' "enthusiasm for innovation".
- Gambro is already producing its own fibers (also for the normal dialysis).
- The Japanese (Asahi, Toray, Teijin) are permanently placing membranes on the market.
- On the one hand filter selling prices are falling and on the other hand fiber costs are increasing.

The planning target has therefore been aimed much higher than at the beginning. It would definitely have been possible to produce a product such as the current Gambro hemofilter one year and a half ago.

But the following specifications were decisive for our development work:

- No momentary successes, but development of basic concepts.
- Learning to spin and no producing.
- Every process step has to be qualified for an economic large-scale production.
- Production has to run fully automatically and continuously (without intermediate handling).
- Minimal manpower requirements.
- No extensive process steps and steps requiring explosion protection.
- The technology also has to be suited for other fibers (normal dialysis).
- It must be possible to quickly boost the production capacity.
- Facilities and equipment will have to be developed and produced by ourselves.

They have to be designed brilliantly simple.

Unfortunately, the last named planning target is a project requirement often being neglected by Fresenius. Many projects broke down in the past because of the estimation that suppliers are running successful complicated developments. It is certainly more comfortable to delegate detailed developments.

If you tax your own brain, it is possible

- to minimize the development risk,
- to design easy systems that are safe for production,
- to save overall, comprehensive but in the end useless specifications and guaranties.

This is certainly only valid for complicated prototype plants.

To sum up, it can be said that we had to reach the high aims with intensive in-house development.'

These development targets definitely include the idea of developing a universal membrane process enabling the production of all dialysis membrane types (low-flux HD, high-flux HD, HF, HDF) only by varying the process parameters. A further key aspect of development was the early orientation to a mass production that is only possible with continuous and fully automatic processes. Remember that, at this time, the volume of today's need for dialysis membranes was unimagined.

Here is a description of the targets for the subsequent realization.

'2. *Project realization*
At the beginning of 1980, a pilot test stand was set up in self-construction being used for pre-tests until the end of the 80s with the aim to gain a planning basis for the manufacturing plant. No process parameters such as

- dosage of spinning media
- spinneret construction
- rinsing time
- drying time
- temperatures
- spinning speeds

were known and however, a facility had to be constructed in detail at the end of 1980 in order to start production. There was no way to use external know-how because either special firms had been detained by producers of cellulose membranes or no equipment could be offered corresponding to our requirements. In addition to that, we envisioned a completely new continuous process being unique to our knowledge.

Despite verification of some process parameters, we certainly had to rely on our technical instinct in many matters and we had to construct into the dark and commission the facility for about 200,000 DM.

Mid 1980 (after only 6 months) the first fiber ran through the facility and we were able to begin the membrane development. From October 1980 until January 1981, I had to stop all operations in order to start the plasma filter production.

After that, there was an intensive work of 12 months on the membrane structure. About 600 spinning tests were run with different spinning compositions and adjustments.

Test and control techniques were developed. The problem "hydrophobicity" took us about 2 months. All involved persons (also Berghof) were of the opinion that the polysulfone fiber was hydrophilic. The reason for the "bogus hydrophilic properties" was the presence of small quantities of solvents and glycerin. It was only Prof. Klein from USA who helped us with this problem on the occasion of his visit.

When studying patent literature, I again and again had the impression of being unprofessional and at the same time bold. How was it possible at that time to draw level with companies such as Asahi, Cordis, Rhône-Poulenc, Enka, etc.? The compositions about polymer chemistry or the like made by highly specialized scientists had a really frustrating effect on us as beginners. We thought that we would never reach this experience gained during decades. But the fact that these works were always contradictory, that they had hardly any theoretical basic concepts and that they rarely led to practical application made me pause. Prof. Klein confirmed this perception.

It appeared that pioneer work can better be performed in smaller companies and that just within the scope of medical technology quantum leaps are still possible with little effort.

In January 1982, we had a membrane that outclassed all other fibers as to its performance data and characteristics. It only had one disadvantage: it was as inhomogeneous as competitive products; that is to say that it also had the notorious pinholes.

Companies such as Asahi, Amicon, and Gambro solved this problem by strongly glycerinizing the fibers and thus making them airtight. Filters could then be checked with air and that worked most of the time. Reports of the hospitals confirmed this "most of the time". We then arrived at the point I mentioned at the beginning: We had to decide whether to enhance development or to copy and quickly place the product on the market? It seemed to be practically impossible to reach such homogeneity.

We tried for 3–4 months and did not get ahead. The great breakthrough only came after a capital investment of about 70,000 DM for an electron microscope approved by Mr. Kröner and Dr. Krick. In August 1982 the unit was set up, at the beginning of November the fiber had the current version and was successfully tested in December.

3. Technical specification of the spinning unit

As already mentioned, a process was realized characterized by homogeneity and continuity, that means that the fiber was rinsed residue-free up from the spinneret with 80 degrees distilled water, dried and collected as completed bundles on a reel. That sounds simple but implied the following problems: In order to remove the complete solvent, a rinsing of 10 minutes was needed resulting in a fiber length of over 300 m regarding the current spinning speed (drying included). Considering today's land prices, such a factory length could hardly be realized. But the installation length could drastically be reduced by reiterating changes in vertical direction. But at this point the problem lied on the part of the rinsing field. We could not find any employees with diving qualification and 80-degrees-temperature resistance. How is it possible to get 50 fibers moving continuously 1 m under the surface of the water and all that with 60 direction changes?

We used a principle that might be unique and I do not want to keep record out of confidentiality reasons (as much as many other details). Anyway, the solution of this problem was the key to a continuous process the main advantages of which are:

- There is no need for a cost-intensive intermediate rinsing made by others for the plasma fiber.
- Repeatable quality is only possible with the same basic conditions. The fiber is completed only after about 5 min. An interrupt of the rinsing process leads to strongly varying fiber qualities. The opinion of Enka and other "experts" that synthetic fibers will never show consistent qualities was completely refuted. The fluctuation range of the filtration performance with different raw material lots was smaller than that of cellulose membranes and had nothing on the plasma fiber.
- Fibers with higher porosity and thus better performance data can be spun, because the tensile strength can be kept low.
- It can be worked without interior liquid preventing a fiber collapsing at intermediate levels.
- Stretching and shrinking of the hollow fibers are kept constant.
- Very low manufacturing costs.
- Special treatments such as crimping can be integrated without problems.

No other works are necessary apart from the dropping off of the finished hollow fiber bundle and the preparation of the spinning solution that is necessary twice per week in case of full production activity. At the moment the facility is running without any difficulty with 8 spinnerets for 2 weeks (also at the weekend); there is only one service person that is already bored.

Capacity:

The system is designed for about 150,000 filters F6 (F60). That requires a doubling of the spinning speed – there have already been experimental tests and apart from some

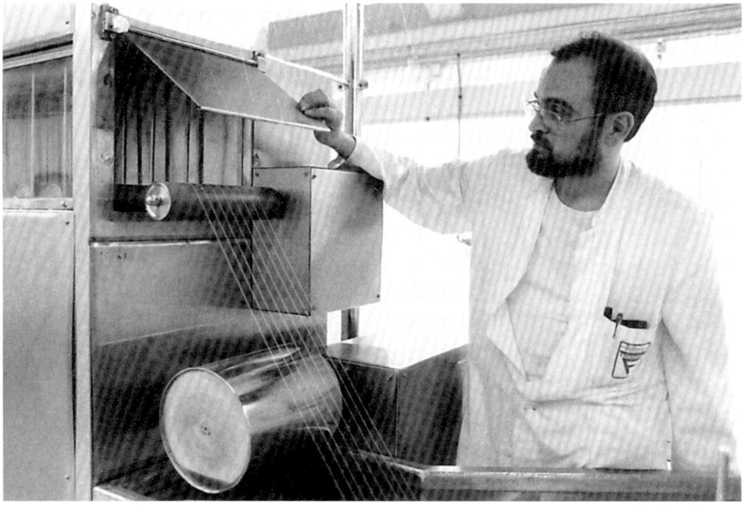

Fig. 1. Elmar Collet produces the first test membranes.

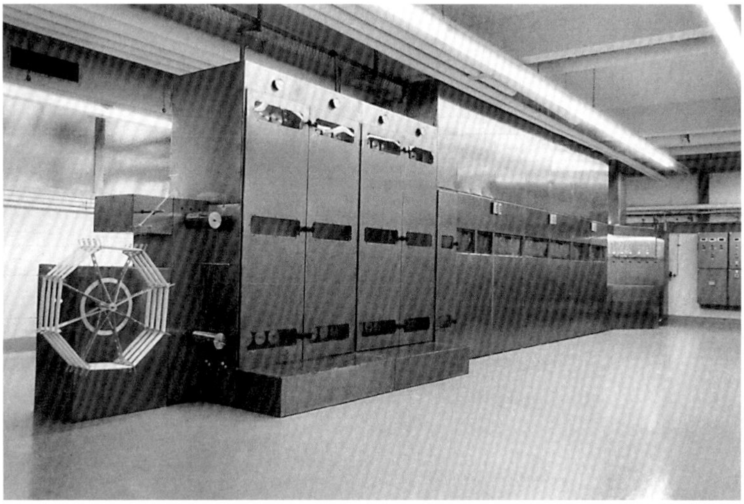

Fig. 2. Fiber spinning pilot test stand mid 1980.

mechanical problems such as roller vibrations because of a too instable bearing no difficulties arose – and an increase of the number of entities from now 8 to 64 spinnerets. This could be realized primitively but quickly by the additional installation of 56 gear pumps (about 25,000 DM). But we want to develop an 8-fold-spinneret (October 1983). However, the problem of a consistent mass distribution means new development effort, but seems answerable to me.

I think that it is necessary to see the systems in order to understand the advantages.

Please find following some pictures that do not reveal details (as shown in figures 1 and 2).'

This section shows that the main focus of innovation was on the technological realization. In the first instance, the process technology engineer was the person being in demand – many detailed solutions had to be found in order to develop a sound, continuous process. Only after implementation of the new solutions where all process conditions were defined and determined as constant in time, was it possible to have a controlled course of the membrane formation mechanism.

'*4. Mechanism of membrane formation*
Take a polymer (e.g. polysulfone), dissolve it in an appropriate solvent, press this honey-like "spinning pulp" through a hole of about 0.3 mm diameter, in the center of which you can find a small tube with an outside diameter of 0.2 mm and an inside diameter of 0.1 mm, send an appropriate coagulant through the inner small tube and drop this partly coagulated hollow fiber in another coagulant (H_2O) and then you have got a hollow fiber. If you are lucky, you can also find some pores in the fiber wall.

This formula is well known and called "dry-wet spinning process". It is based on the physical process of the fast running phase inversion that means that the fiber freezes at a special solvent-coagulant concentration. The concentration change activating the precipitation procedure is caused by the diffusion of solvents and coagulants running at the same time. Because of the manifold interacting process parameters (temperatures, precipitation speed, spinning speed, concentrations, proportions, molecular masses) these processes are extraordinarily complex even for a textile fiber without pores, hard to handle and can only be gotten under control by empirical tests.

If you want to achieve and maintain a special pore structure and distribution (pore diameter of 10–50 nm), this will be the point at which every theory ends. Then you can only follow your gut instinct.

An example: If we change a concentration theoretically by 2%, we will get a cascade filter instead of a hemofilter. At the same time the spinning speed must be increased because of the slower precipitation. This leads to an increased mass supply. Thereby the concentration at the phase boundary and thus the pore formation change. Therefore the inner liquid also has to be varied – results in an even higher spinning speed – and thus you are deadlocked if you do not additionally vary the air gap height further boosting the complexity.

Today we developed a certain feeling for spinning enabling us to predict certain settings. But the first tests were more than frustrating, so that I realized why Enka had been unrivaled for such a long time.

Today we are also able to spin other polymers under the same procedure. For example, in the meantime, we made a test with our Makrolon (polycarbonate). Surprisingly, we got the same performance data.'

This is a simple description of the dry-wet spinning process for the production of polysulfone membranes. In fact, it is quite easy to produce any membrane based on this formula and one even does not need luck to get some pores. However, it also becomes apparent that it is difficult to achieve specified properties due to complex influences and interrelationships. Today, these influences have been researched better and, based on this knowledge, it is now possible to

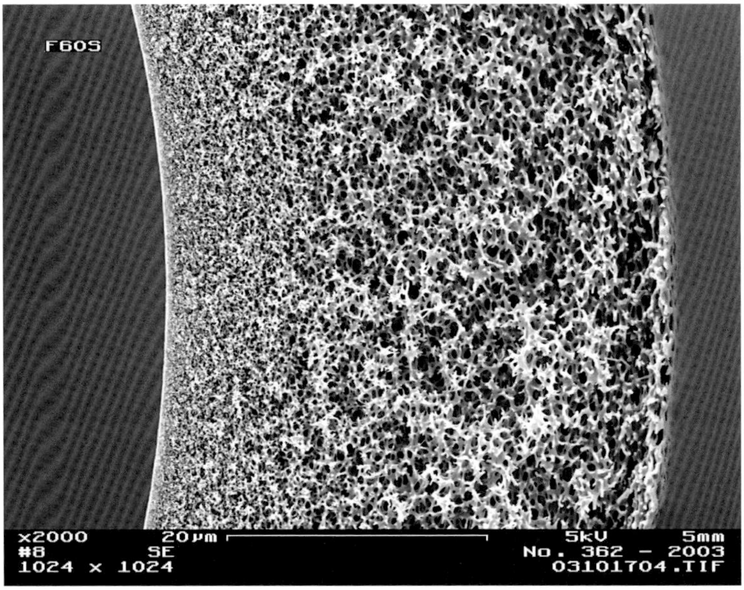

Fig. 3. SEM image of the polysulfone membrane, cross section of the asymmetrical membrane wall. ×2,000.

produce any membrane with any pore size of 1 nm to 1 μm and thus to cover the whole field of blood purification therapies. Pore sizes of 50 nm are well suited for convective therapies as these membranes already retain albumin to a great extent.

'5. Advantages of the hollow fiber "PS 600"

At the beginning of the project the aim was: "Production of a hemofiltration fiber similar to Gambro or Amicon". The mass transport is purely convective with these relatively thick-walled capillaries (80 μ). We were of the opinion that these wall thicknesses strongly limit the diffusive mass transport. Employees of the company Berghof completely excluded diffusive clearance, because then it would be necessary to work with wall thicknesses of 8–12 μ, as with Cuprophan. At a certain project phase, we had the idea to verify this expert opinion. The result with this 35 μ membrane was striking. The purely diffusive clearance for B_{12} was 1.5-fold higher than for the 8 μ membrane of Enka for our "D 6". The reason for this phenomenon seeming to be inexplicable at first sight is the following: The composition of the wall is extremely asymmetrical, that is to say that the smallest and thus limiting pores lie on the internal side of the hollow fiber in a coat being about 0.5 μ thick. The remaining pores are becoming greater and greater from inside to outside and are only forming a supporting layer that is hardly able to resist diffusion because of its high porosity.

However, the Cuprophan membranes (also Cordis, Toray, Teijin, Asahi cellulose) are constructed symmetrically and therefore substances have to "fight" their way through a porous wall of 8–12 μ.

This perception which was new for us completely changed the goal. If we succeeded to outrival the D 6 – accepted as the best hemodiafilter – with our own fibers, this would open an additional market for about 50,000 filters.

The second part of this report documents the advantage of our new type F 60, the high-performance data is reached with only 1.3 m^2 (!) compared to 2.0 m^2 for the D 6 (Cuprophan membrane with a wall thickness of 10 μm).

As already mentioned, a further advantage of the new fiber lies in the absolutely constant structure enabling a bubble point test.

This uniform pore structure has another great advantage. For the range of fluctuation is very small, we could adjust the pore diameter very large without running the risk of the passage of albumin.

This can practically be seen in the steep cut-off almost resembling the human kidney (part 2). The high inulin clearance can also be explained thereby.

Because of the new test method it is also not necessary any more to "cram" the membrane with glycerin. Last year, Asahi set its PAN membrane more open-pored. But therefore they were forced to even more glycerinize – in parts the fiber is almost transparent. The problems with blood leaks followed immediately.

Our "dry" fiber can be stored and processed without any difficulties (not hygroscopic).'

The hemocompatibility aspect of the membranes (which is much better than that of cellulose membranes) remained unmentioned up to this point because this was not known at that time. However, given that the membrane with its 1–2 m^2 represents the greatest artificial material surface in the extracorporeal circuit, hemocompatibility is a very important characteristic of the membrane material. Polysulfone is characterized by a very low activation of the coagulation and complement systems as well as by a lower interaction with blood cells. It is also steam sterilizable, which contributes further to its good hemocompatibility profile. The optimal pore size of a dialysis membrane always presents a compromise between sufficient retention of blood proteins and maximum permeability for toxins. For the retention of albumin and other higher-molecular proteins, it is completely sufficient to arrange a separation layer, consisting of one single layer of small and preferably identical pores that is mechanically supported by a highly-porous substrate layer. Here this was achieved in an almost optimal way: the polysulfone membrane has a separation layer of about 200 nm with a very tight pore size distribution and a substrate layer with a porosity of about 50% so that, in this layer, diffusing molecules barely meet resistance. Because the developed technology enabled an absolutely constant process control and thus a zero-defect membrane with stable properties, a very high cut-off could be chosen when adjusting the membrane. Thus a considerable increase in efficiency was also possible for a hemodialysis membrane with purely diffusive transport. Due to the lack of defects, this was the first synthetic membrane that could be tested using the bubble point test. The diffusive transport could further be improved by the invention of fiber curling: here the concentration gradient as driving force for diffusion was increased by the improved dialysate flow around the fibers.

‘6. *Post-processing*
If there is a disadvantage of the new fiber to Cuprophan at all, it can only theoretically be the less tensile strength of about 25 g (8 μ Cuprophan – 40 g). That means that the fiber cannot be interwoven anymore and our specific product advantage "homogeneous dialysate distribution" would be inapplicable. There were actually big problems to get a good fluid flow. We tried strong crossing at the reel, but the result was not easily repeatable.

Toray spirally wraps two hollow fibers with an additional multiphilic textile fiber – an enormous effort.

We had a better idea. The fibers are slightly crimped with a very simple device (curler) in an inline process.

The results were amazing. Dialysate distribution and thus the clearance were better (!) than that of our hemoflow series that means that by this trick the assumed disadvantage turned out to be an advantage.

At the same time, the very labor intensive spooling could be saved. The bundles will directly be inserted into the housing. However, PU potting has to be executed at a bundle in a centrifuge procedure. The following production steps are the same as those of hemoflow. An additional test console is integrated in the end rinsing.

7. Perspectives and next steps
The version "F 60" will definitely be a fast seller and will result in a positive gross margin by the way. But in 1983, hemofiltration and hemodiafiltration represent an interesting but also limited market of about 150,000 units.

It will indeed be possible to use the "F 60" with our machine 2008 and other machines with a balancing system for the normal dialysis but unfortunately, the vast majority of machines are non-balancing machines.

The system 2008 and "F 60" would nevertheless be the best normal dialysis currently existing (statement of Dr. Streicher). It would definitely be a good idea to merchandise it because this would lead to an enormous increase in machine sales.

Although the future almost certainly belongs to the "open-pored membrane" in combination with machines with a balancing system, the main business is the normal dialysis with low ultrafiltration performance.

Based on this fact, we made some spinning tests in December to get fibers with low UF. The aim was to get similar performance data to the "G 1" Enka fiber having the leading position at the moment. We only changed one spinning parameter and achieved a surprising success. In calendar week 4 we will produce fibers and at the beginning of February we will perform clinical tests with "F 6".

I believe devoutly to the success.’

The high variability of the developed membrane production process also created a reasonable economic basis for successful market penetration. In 1983, the market for hemofiltration and HDF membranes was still very limited. However, the production lines operated at full capacity producing membranes for the evolving high-flux hemodialysis and for low-flux dialysis, which was the standard at that time. Thus, products for convective therapies could also be offered at acceptable prices.

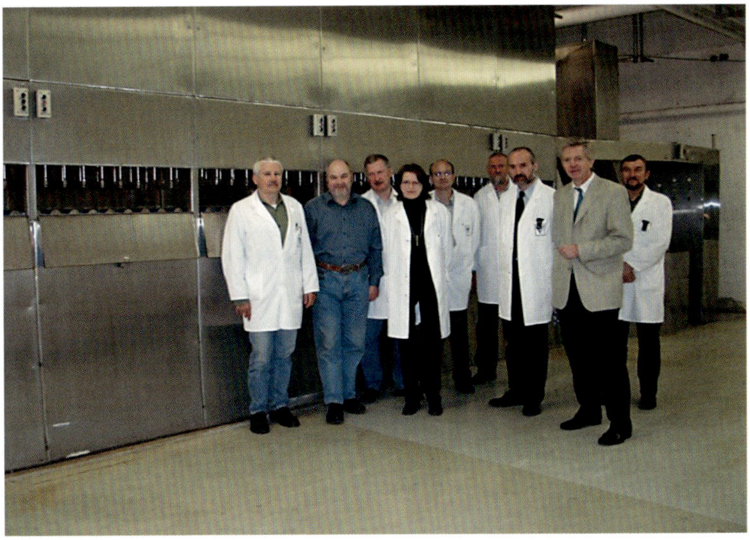

Fig. 4. The polysulfone development team: Rainer Meyer, Walter Guth, Erwin Franiek, Ellen Krug, Elmar Collet, Hans-Gerd Fehr, Ulrich Kramp, Klaus Heilmann, Hans-Josef Lambert (Bernd Nederlof is not in the photo; photograph taken in 2002 at the closure of the pilot plant).

'8. *Concluding remark*

When taking stock, the reasons of the project success are not to be forgotten. I mean that people are always responsible.

If Dr. Krick had not given me a great leeway for decisions and had not had the courage to take risks, the project would have collapsed at an early stage.

In my opinion, the risk always lies in the perfect solution of details.

At this point I want to present the members of the project team. It goes without saying that they worked more and harder to achieve this pioneer work and that they spent some leisure time. But the key success factor for the project was that they did not realize their work as work, nobody was able to escape the fascination of the project despite some huge setbacks.

Mr. Kramp was the technical project leader and responsible for plant engineering together with Mr. Guth. The plant itself is the best documentation for the quality of their work. Mr. Franiek and Mrs. Krug were responsible for the chemical and physical tests. Without Mr. Franiek's consulting the progress especially in the chemical-physical field would not have been possible.

Even Prof. Klein was impressed by the extraordinary preparation technologies and outstanding fiber pictures being part of the field of responsibility of Mrs. Krug in addition to other tests.

Mr. Collet operated the spinning plant and made all spinning tests. There was no admittance even for me in case susceptible settings were made and sometimes this was definitely a good solution for I am known to set people's nerves on edge.

St. Wendel, 20th January 1983

K. Heilmann'

The fundamentals of polysulfone dialysis membranes were therefore established, but the development proceeded further with aims to improve the product performance and to adjust product quantities to meet increasing demand, thus improving the quality of the membranes and reducing production cost. The controllable lack of defects in polysulfone membranes is a precondition for the absolute retention of endotoxins. A pyrogen-free substitution fluid can be produced at the dialysis machine by filtration through such a membrane. For this purpose, dialysate is filtered through another polysulfone membrane filter and is then available as substitution solution for HDF. Consequently, today the polysulfone membrane also enables on-line HDF.

Torsten Keller
Fresenius Medical Care Deutschland GmbH
Membrane & Filter Development
Frankfurter Strasse 6–8, DE–66606 St. Wendel (Germany)
Tel. +49 6851 807 407, E-Mail torsten.keller@fmc-ag.com

Krick G, Ronco C (eds): On-Line Hemodiafiltration: The Journey and the Vision.
Contrib Nephrol. Basel, Karger, 2011, vol 175, pp 27–34

The Machine and the Therapy Concept

R.N. Greenwood

Lister Renal Unit, Stevenage, UK

Abstract

Maintenance haemodialysis became established in mainstream clinical practice in the 1960s. For pragmatic reasons, diffusive dialysis was the technique which underpinned its success. Over the next 15 years it was shown that short- and medium-term survival depended only on a critical level of urea clearance being achieved. Uncomplicated technology with negligible capacity for middle molecule removal could deliver this and the case for developing more sophisticated machines able to broaden the spectrum of solute removal was unconvincing. Dialysis-related amyloidosis which was recognised in the mid-1980s as a devastating complication in long survivors disturbed this complacency. The journey to develop machines which could deliver broad-spectrum solute removal while exposing patients only to ultrapure fluids and biocompatible materials is described elsewhere in this text. The Lister Renal Unit was established in 1988. A fruitful collaboration between the multidisciplinary clinical team and engineering colleagues in the R&D Department of Fresenius contributed to a steady and in-depth understanding of the effect of superimposing convection on diffusive dialysis. From the outset only high-flux dialysis using ultrapure fluids was employed. Haemodiafiltration (HDF) was introduced in 1993. This paper summarises our observations regarding the relative contributions of natural renal function and convective blood purification to long-term outcomes. We have recently reported a 19-year experience which has allowed us to more clearly define the rationale for HDF in modern clinical practice. HDF is an engineering triumph which is likely to universally supersede diffusive dialysis. The challenge for clinicians moving forward is to learn in which treatment schedules this technology can best be deployed to improve the health prospects of patients with kidney failure.

Diffusive Dialysis in the 1960s and 1970s

In developing apparatus for maintenance blood purification, reproducing the function of the human kidney, which is a dominantly convective process, was

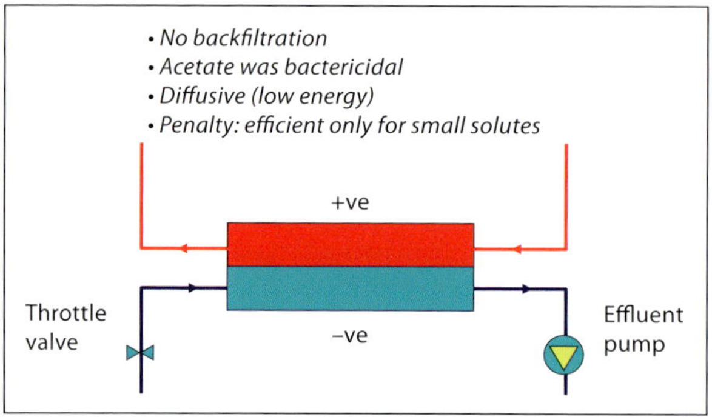

Fig. 1. Dialysis machine design in the 1970s.

probably seriously considered. Glomerular filtration rate (GFR) is approximately 100 ml/min which totals 150 litres/day of which approximately 147 litres are reabsorbed by active metabolic tubular function – a high-energy process requiring a renal blood flow rate of approximately 1.2 litres/min, a quarter of cardiac output, being taken by the kidneys. To mimic such a process in the 1960s would have been thwarted by several factors. First, there was no suitable membrane with the appropriate hydraulic permeability, the cost of replacing filtered fluid with sterile replacement fluid would have been prohibitively expensive and, much more daunting, the huge blood flow necessary to achieve this level of filtration in intermittent therapy could not be accessed from the circulation. The inevitable outcome was a diffusive system. It was fortuitous that a relatively inexpensive cellulosic membrane was available with good diffusive properties and a convenient level of hydraulic permeability which allowed a manageable amount of ultrafiltration to take place during a 6–10 h session while employing only modest transmembrane pressures. The basic laws of physics dictate that such low energy expenditure in a diffusive system would come with a cost – the inability to move large molecules from blood no matter how porous the membrane. Diffusive dialysis could only be a weak imitation of the depurative quality of natural renal function.

It is worth considering the features which enabled the simple design of early dialysis machines to be safe in clinical practice (fig. 1). Approximately 1 m^2 of cellulosic membrane was used in a flat-plate configuration. Blood was pushed in a thin film between two membrane sheets and dialysis fluid was pulled across the other side of these 'flat plates' by an effluent pump in countercurrent flow. Across the whole 1 m^2 membrane area there was positive pressure between blood and dialysate ensuring no prospect of dialysate entering the bloodstream. Acetate, which was used as an easily metabolised substitute for bicarbonate, was bactericidal. These features combined to ensure that the risks from infection from impure dialysis fluids were largely restricted to the processes of reassembling the Kiil dialyzer and the re-use procedures which were in common usage at the time.

Coming across a kidney machine first in 1978, the author observed a surprisingly unsophisticated system which looked messy and poorly engineered. From the medical point of view, it was perplexing how such a system of diffusion could reverse the symptoms of uraemia and return patients to good health (except for profound anaemia) while only small molecules were being removed from uraemic plasma.

However, clinical experience did not fit this dubious theoretical construct. The first randomised controlled trial in dialysis – the National Cooperative Dialysis Study (NCDS, 1980) – showed that a critical level of urea clearance was all that was needed for complication-free survival. The effect was noticeable by 3 months. Although the pioneering work which had been taking place in the USA [1] and in Germany at the University Hospital in Giessen [2] a few years earlier was inspiring, the overwhelming opinion of the nephrology community, was that the problems of dialysis were mostly solved and there was no need to pursue more complex technical solutions, particularly any involving expensive replacement solutions. In any case, continuous ambulatory peritoneal dialysis (CAPD) appeard as an additional bridge to transplant rather than maintenance HD. Energies became more focused on how to accommodate an expanding dialysis population in cash-strapped healthcare systems rather than on the dialysis technique itself.

Design Changes

Attending the EDTA meeting in Prague in 1980 the author observed the introduction of volumetric control of dialysis fluid with some concern. By that time there had been very significant advances in the design of dialyzers now being produced in capillary form with exciting new membranes, in particular polysulfone and polyamide. While volumetric control for ultrafiltration was necessary when using membranes with high permeability, it was clear that some of the advantages of the traditional circuit (above) would be lost. The rigid movement of dialysis fluid would almost inevitably result in infusion of dialysate into blood, which looked risky in terms of endotoxin transfer. Again, clinical experience did not fit with this theoretical construct. It appeared that 'backfiltration' did not have any clinical sequelae in an era when microbiological standards for dialysis fluid were lax. With the benefit of hindsight, this could have been explained by the excellent absorptive barriers of these membranes to microbiological transfer.

In retrospect, rigid volumetric control of dialysis fluid provided an ideal platform for the manipulation of dialysis fluid flow – the engineering starting point for the modern haemodiafiltration (HDF) machine.

The Emerging Case for Added Convection – 'Diafiltration'

For clinicians working in the UK NHS in the early 1980s, the challenges centred around more resources to create dialysis spaces, the liberalisation of acceptance of patients onto dialysis, vascular access problems, the continuing poor results of transplantation and the perpetual battle against profound anaemia. Little attention seemed to be focussed on the dialysis technique itself. All this changed in 1985 with the recognition of dialysis-related amyloidosis. Patients had been complaining for some time about symptoms of carpal tunnel syndrome and 'frozen shoulders'. First referred to as dialysis arthropathy, it was re-named more specifically as dialysis-related amyloidosis after biopsies of synovial tissue revealed deposition of long chain proteins which seemed to be preferentially deposited in joints. A short time later the building block of this particular amyloid was identified as β_2-microglobulin (β2M) which was found on the surface of most nucleated cells in the body. With a molecular weight of 11,500 there was no prospect of significant removal by diffusive dialysis.

There was more to it than this. Shaldon with a small group of enthusiasts in Europe put forward the 'interleukin hypothesis', which suggested that intimate exposure of blood to bacterial endotoxin across 'incompatible' membranes made dialysis a pro-inflammatory process which prompted the release of cytokines from circulating monocytes. It was repetitive inflammation which encouraged the deposition of β2M in joints, aided by high circulated levels. Those involved in dialysis had a new challenge. Firstly, much more attention would have to be paid to the purity of dialysis fluid. Also more attention would have to be paid to the biocompatibility of dialysis membranes. Finally, there was a direct clinical reason rather than a theoretical one to pursue the convective removal of middle molecules.

Engineers in the dialysis industry had a good starting point. At their disposal was a proven system for volumetric control of dialysis fluid and new membranes such as polysulfone, which not only had excellent diffusive and convective properties, but were also effective barriers to transfer of microbiological contaminants from dialysis fluid into blood. However, the intelligent use of these materials to develop machines that could provide broad-spectrum solute removal within the strict confines of healthcare budgets was a huge challenge. What took place over the next few years is articulated elsewhere in this book.

Engineering and Clinic Collaboration

In 1988 a new kidney service was established with an estimated catchment population of about 1.1 million people centred in Stevenage, which is 35 miles north of London. While at Barts Hospital in London there had been some contact with the R&D team at Fresenius in Bad Homburg, but shortly before the opening of the Lister Renal Unit (LRU) a meeting took place with Hans Polaschegg to discuss a possible cooperation between clinicians and engineers in the development of new ideas. Although the precedent had long been set for cooperation between clinicians and pharmaceutical companies, this was forward thinking from a technology company. From the outset, the LRU would have a commitment to biomedical engineering developments and the arrangement provided a valuable opportunity for R&D engineers led by Hans Polaschegg and assisted by Thomas Roy to have access to the clinical environment. At one point there were more engineers and computer people employed in the LRU than nurses. The former included Colin Aldridge and a young Paul Chamney. Matthias Kramer was a regular collaborator.

From the outset, high-flux membranes, chiefly polysulfone, were used in all patients. Experience with online HDF dated from about 1992. Much investment was made in bacteriological surveillance of dialysis water and substitution fluid. Rigorous test schedules were developed.

At that time there was acute awareness of the emergence of clinical standards for dialysis which came chiefly from the USA in response to the poor outcomes in HD. In order to protect patients from the risks associated with reducing dialysis times which was taking place in the USA and then across Europe, the LRU enthusiastically embraced urea kinetic modelling as a means to ensure that adequate doses of dialysis were delivered either by high-flux dialysis or HDF. Dr. James Tattersall was a founder member of the LRU. His pioneering work in kinetic modelling, which furthered the understanding of the impact of natural kidney function on health and survival of patients on CAPD and HD, was highly valued. In the mid-1990s my close colleague, Dr. Ken Farrington, assumed a leadership role in the clinical research programme. In the last few years, researchers at the LRU have reported a 19-year experience with high-flux dialysis and HDF. HDF has become the preferred modality for all patients, our ability to deliver this for all being constrained only by the finances available. HDF is favoured for patients who have lost natural kidney function and who tend to have a high muscle mass. The next few paragraphs summarise the main clinical findings over nearly two decades of observation.

Natural Residual Renal Function and HDF

The classical form of urea kinetic modelling as described by Frank Gotch and John Sargent recognises the contributions of both dialysis and residual renal function (RRF) to overall dialysis dose. One of our first observations was that the initiation of dialysis has no effect whatsoever on the decline in natural kidney function, be it in CAPD patients or in high-flux dialysis/HDF [3]. This was in contrast to many prior studies which had suggested that HD, unlike CAPD, leads to rapid decline in RRF. We concluded that, just as RRF is an important determinant of the health and indeed the survival of patients on peritoneal dialysis, the same is also likely to apply to patients on HD.

A study comparing the use of high-flux polysulfone membranes with low-flux polysulfone and cellulosic membranes concluded that it was flux, not biocompatibility, which determined β2M levels. It became apparent in the mid-1990s that amyloidosis had virtually disappeard and no longer seemed to be an long-term outcome after 10 years on dialysis. It is likely that the accumulation of β2M itself was not the cause of amyloidosis, which vindicated somewhat Shaldon's views about the inflammatory nature of dialysis related to water quality. The disappearance of dialysis amyloid was probably driven chiefly by adherence to standards which had been set for the microbiological purity of dialysis fluids.

C-reactive protein (CRP) is a routine laboratory test which found a place into routine clinical practice in the mid-1990s as a very useful marker of systemic inflammation. We observed CRP levels in our dialysis patients over a number of years and although there were many 'spikes' recorded in many patients, the vast majority of these could be explained by discrete clinical events and did not seem to relate to the dialytic process itself. Essentially, patients on high-flux dialysis and HDF did not experience inflammation, at least as identified by routine temperature and CRP estimations. As has been pointed out by Thomas Roy, it was necessary to overcome some of the fears that had been perpetuated about the potential for inflammation using on-line technology. It is the author's view that this fear has now been firmly put to rest. This is a tribute to the innovation of sequential filtration and the refinement of pre-dialysis tests for filter integrity in ensuring purity of dialysis fluid and HDF replacement fluid.

The contribution of RRF to overall 'renal replacement' in dialysis patients is illustrated in figure 2. At the LRU, mean GFR at dialysis initiation is 8.7 ml/min as measured by creatinine clearance. On average, RRF continues to make a useful contribution for up to 5 years. At dialysis initiation, GFR equates to about 87 litres/week convection. A patient on HDF would experience about 60 litres/week of added convection over the basic diffusive process – a similar order of magnitude.

RRF is powerful. We have observed that higher intradialytic ultrafiltration rates are required in patients who have a residual urea clearance (KrU) <1 ml/min [4]. Whilst this might seem intuitively obvious, it is an important observation since DOPPS data shows us that a high ultrafiltration rate carries a significant risk. Patients with KrU >2 ml/min have superior phosphate control. This is important since high serum phosphate is also associated with increased mortality risk in HD patients.

Patients with KrU <2 ml/min have a higher erythropoietin resistance index, which may reflect increased uraemic toxicity in patients who have lost their residual kidney function. Patients who have KrU >1 ml/min at 3 months

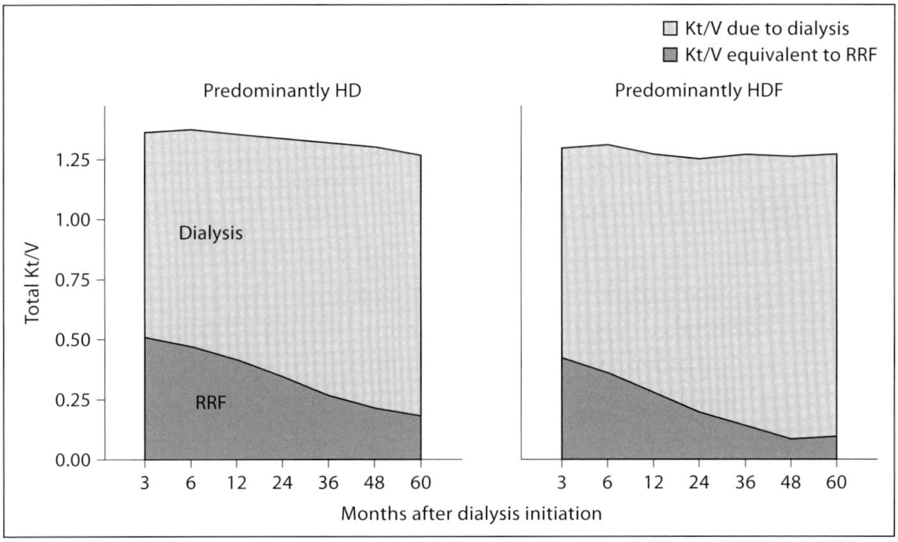

Fig. 2. Contributions of dialysis and RRF.

following dialysis initiation have an improved survival over those patients who are oliguric. The presence of RRF therefore seems to be a strong predictor of wellbeing and possibly survival in dialysis patients.

Clinical Rationale for HDF

In our patients, β2M levels increase with dialysis vintage and as natural renal function declines. These trends are observed in patients receiving high-flux dialysis or HDF. RRF is the major determinant of β2M levels. However, in patients who become oliguric, HDF has measurable superiority over high-flux dialysis in abrogating further rises in β2M levels [5]. It is justifiable to propose that HDF provides superior replacement of lost natural kidney function than high-flux dialysis.

The rationale for HDF is therefore strongest in patients who have the greatest potential for a long-term survival and in patients who have lost natural renal function. It is worth noting that patients who choose home HD are generally constituents of this group. Patients who have failed on peritoneal dialysis are often in this group as are those who are highly sensitised and experience a long wait for transplantation or those who have rejected several transplants.

HDF is clearly an evolutionary milestone in dialytic blood purification. While doctors have often agonised over evidence to justify change in practice our engineering colleagues seem to have been less constrained and moved ahead to develop the most logical way to purify blood using currently available materials. In the case of HD, this has been cleverly executed and an improved 'broad-spectrum' blood purification therapy has been provided to users whilst remaining within the constraints of reimbursement.

The author recognises the managerial firmness of purpose of Dr. Gatti and colleagues which must have been necessary to overcome regulatory approval hurdles and to encourage R&D over such a long time-scale. As clinicians we applaud the decision made to incorporate HDF as the standard feature of operation of the Fresenius 5008 which would no longer be regarded as an optional extra. To the author's knowledge, no depletion syndromes have been identified whilst employing broad-spectrum solute removal. There seems very little justification therefore in continuing to administer diffusive HD as a routine treatment. 'HDF is common sense'.

References

1 Leber HW, Wizemann V, Techert F: Simultaneous hemofiltration/hemodialysis: short- and long-term tolerance. Introduction of a system for automatic fluid replacement. Artif Organs 1980;4:108–112.

2 Henderson LW, Sanfelippo ML, Beans E: 'On-line' preparation of sterile pyrogen-free electrolyte solution. Trans Am Soc Artif Intern Organs 1978;24:465–467.

3 McKane W, Chandna SM, Tattersall JE, Greenwood RN, Farrington K: Identical decline of residual renal function in high-flux biocompatible hemodialysis and CAPD. Kidney Int 2002;61:256–265.

4 Vilar E, Fry AC, Wellstead D, Tattersall JE, Greenwood RN, Farrington K: Long-term outcomes in online haemodiafiltration and high-flux haemodialysis: a comparative analysis. Clin J Am Soc Nephrol 2009;4:1944–1953.

5 Fry AC, Singh DK, Chandna SM, Farrington K: Relative Importance of residual renal function and convection in determining β_2-microglobulin levels in high-flux haemodialysis and online haemodiafiltration. Blood Purif 2007:25:295–302.

Dr. R.N. Greenwood
Lister Renal Unit, Coreys Mill Lane
Stevenage SG1 4AB (UK)
Tel. +44 1438 781157
E-Mail dr.greenwood.home@virgin.net

Krick G, Ronco C (eds): On-Line Hemodiafiltration: The Journey and the Vision.
Contrib Nephrol. Basel, Karger, 2011, vol 175, pp 35–45

Backfiltration: Past, Present and Future

Armando Vazquez Rangel · Jeong Chul Kim ·
Manish Kaushik · Francesco Garzotto · Mauro Neri ·
Dinna N. Cruz · Claudio Ronco

Department of Nephrology, San Bortolo Hospital and International Renal Research Institute
Vicenza (IRRIV), Vicenza, Italy

Abstract

Backfiltration has been recognized to be present in most diffusive-convective therapies. Although initially considered an inconvenience due to its implications in transport of contaminants in dialysate to the blood compartment, the availability of ultrapure dialysate has prompted a fresh look at the phenomenon of backfiltration with the possibility of exploiting it to further enhance the convective clearance of middle and large molecules. This review discusses the historical aspects of backfiltration, its mechanisms and influencing factors, and subsequently the different hemodialysis techniques in relation to increasing or diminishing this phenomenon.

Backtransport in a hollow-fiber hemodialyzer is defined as the movement of water and substances from the dialysate to the blood. This includes two mechanisms: (1) backdiffusion: movement of substances along a concentration gradient, and (2) backfiltration: a convective mechanism dependent upon the local pressure gradient across the membrane. This gradient, called transmembrane pressure (TMP), is defined by the formula:

$$TMP = P_b - (P_d + \pi_b),$$

where P_b is the hydrostatic pressure in the blood, P_d is the hydrostatic pressure in dialysate, and π_b is the oncotic pressure in blood. When TMP is positive, the hydraulic flow is from the blood to the dialysate side (filtration); nevertheless, if at any point the TMP becomes negative, backfiltration occurs [1]. This constitutes a dynamic process along the filter, where factors related to patient characteristics, dialysis prescription, filters and membranes properties,

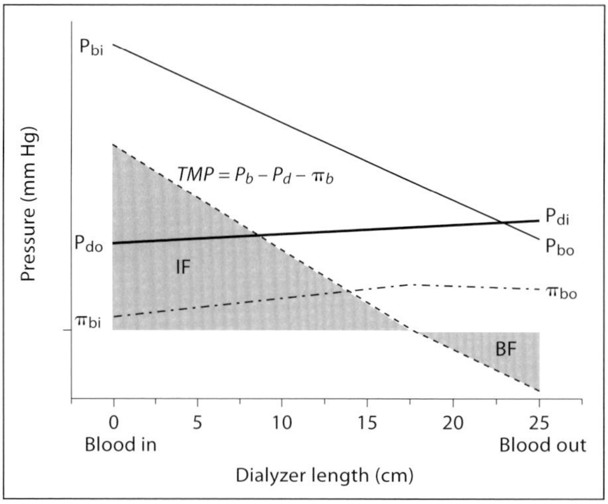

Fig. 1. Pressure profiles along the dialyzer contributing to internal filtration (IF) and backfiltration (BF). TMP = Transmembrane pressure; P_{bi} = inlet hydrostatic blood pressure; P_{bo} = outlet blood pressure; P_{di} = inlet hydrostatic dialysate pressure; P_{do} = outlet dialysate pressure; π_{bi} = inlet oncotic blood pressure; π_{bo} = outlet oncotic blood pressure.

and dialysis modality, play a role in promoting or ameliorating backfiltration. Basically, starting with a high hydrostatic pressure in the blood compartment, the filtration process is favored in the proximal part of the filter; this happens in proportion to the ultrafiltration (UF) rate allowed by the membrane. This initial UF, together with the geometrical properties of the fibers, will produce a hydrostatic pressure drop in the blood compartment along the filter, promoting hemoconcentration and a consequent progressive increase in the oncotic pressure. Both factors reduce the TMP in the distal part of the filter and, together with the incoming dialysate pressure, can contribute to backfiltration (fig. 1).

While backtransport of chemical impurities and microorganisms from contaminated dialysate to the blood compartment has been a concern since the inception of hemodialysis (HD), the existence of backfiltration during high-flux HD was first empirically demonstrated by Schmidt et al. [2]. These investigators showed that the dialysate inflow hydraulic pressure did indeed exceed the blood outlet hydraulic pressure minus the blood outlet oncotic pressure, establishing the existence of this driving force. Therefore, having a higher pressure in the blood compartment is not enough to prevent backfiltration, since the oncotic pressure in the blood plays a major role possibly starting from the second third of the filter.

Direct measurements of backfiltration are few. Leypoldt et al. [3] developed a method for determining backfiltration rates by measuring the changes in local concentrations of a marker molecule along the dialyzer length. Ronco [4], on the hand, measured radiolabeled albumin macroaggregates added to the blood using a gamma camera. The increase in marker macromolecule concentration indicated internal filtration, and a decrease indicated backfiltration.

Historical Importance of Backfiltration

Clinical appreciation of this entity regained importance with the evolution from using predominantly diffusive clearance to using mixed diffusive-convective clearance with higher permeability membranes. In an attempt to improve clearance of middle and large molecules, and reduce bioincompatibility, modified cellulose and eventually asymmetrical thick-walled synthetic membranes were developed. These membranes exhibit higher solute and water permeability (β_2-microglobulin clearance >20 ml/min and UF coefficient >20 ml/h/mm Hg) [5–7], which by themselves increased the risk of backfiltration of endotoxins and bacteria from suboptimal quality dialysate. Besides, with the reintroduction of bicarbonate buffered dialysate in the 1980s (justified by better blood pressure and cardiopulmonary outcomes compared to acetate-based dialysate), an increased risk of contamination and pyrogenic reactions was observed. The reason is that bicarbonate solution is an excellent medium for propagation of bacteria [8, 9].

Clinical impact of backfiltration became evident from observations of these pyrogenic reactions in high-flux HD patients, the incidence of which was directly proportional to the degree of dialysate contamination [10]. Antibodies specific to dialysate-derived endotoxins have been more commonly identified in high-flux HD than in low-flux HD patients [11]. Laude-Sharp et al. [12] first demonstrated in vitro the passage into the blood compartment of intact lipopolysaccharides capable of inducing IL-1 in dialyzers with acrylonitrile, polysulfone and cuprophan membranes. Panichi et al. [13] evaluated the long-term effects of backfiltration on cytokine production in a multi-center study. They demonstrated that post/pre ratios of IL-1 receptor antagonist and IL-1β were higher in patients receiving hemodiafiltration (HDF) with backfiltration compared to those on HDF without backfiltration.

In context of the above, the use of ultrapure dialysate is a prerequisite for the safe delivery of mixed diffusive-convective therapies with high water permeability membranes. The minimum quality requirement of dialysate as defined by ISO standards is <100 CFU/ml for viable microbial count and <0.5 EU/ml for endotoxin concentration [14], while the ERA-EDTA best practice guidelines and Swedish Pharmacopoeia have stricter definitions for the endotoxin levels (<0.25 EU/ml) [15]. For ultrapure dialysate, the definition has been established as <0.1 CFU/ml for bacteria and as <0.03 EU/ml for endotoxins [14].

Patients treated with ultrapure dialysis fluid have shown a decrease in serum β_2-microglobulin concentrations and related amyloidosis, a decrease in markers of inflammatory response and oxidant stress, an increased responsiveness to erythropoietin, better preservation of residual renal function, and improved nutritional status [14, 16]. These observations have led to the recommendation that ultrapure dialysis fluid should be used for high-flux HD, although it has been recognized that obtaining this level of purity on a routine basis might not yet be feasible in all dialysis settings [14, 16].

A practical approach to achieve good water quality has been to equip dialysis machines with polysulfone ultrafilters as part of the water treatment process [17, 18]. In vitro studies have shown that polysulfone membranes have considerable capacity to adsorb pyrogens from contaminated dialysate [19]. Ronco et al. [17] have explained this adsorption by the interaction of negatively charged lipopolysaccharide with hydrophobic domains of these membranes.

Factors Influencing Backfiltration

As previously mentioned, backfiltration is directly determined by pressures in the blood and dialysate compartments. Pressures at the inlet and outlet of the blood compartment are mostly dependent on the speed of the blood pump and the resistance of the filter. The latter is directly influenced by the number, length and inner radius of the fibers, and the viscosity of blood associated with the water permeability of the membrane [20].

Water Permeability

In low water permeability membranes, the lower total internal filtration might not produce the required drop in TMP for backfiltration to occur. However, in high permeability membranes, the higher water total internal filtration generates a more significant drop in hydrostatic pressure and a more pronounced hemoconcentration raising the oncotic pressure. This results in a lower TMP in the second half of the filter and consequent backfiltration by 'oncotic flux'. This last process could be self-limited since the amount of water entering from the dialysate to the blood decreases the oncotic and increases the hydrostatic pressures. But given the actual use of volume control systems in HD machines, the restriction in net UF generates an increase in hydrostatic pressure in the dialysate, and therefore a higher degree of backfiltration. This 'convective flux' overrides the self-limiting mechanism of the 'oncotic flux' [20]. In this sense, low UF or absence thereof does not avoid internal filtration using high water permeability membranes; moreover, if this filtered plasma water does not match a corresponding UF rate, backfiltration will be produced. This leads to the concept of critical or obligate UF as the minimum required UF rate to avoid backfiltration [21].

Experimental modifications have been described to manipulate water permeability. While membranes might not show the same permeability to water flux in both directions because of the formation of a protein layer, new membranes could be designed having low resistance for water towards the dialysate but high resistance towards the blood compartment [20]. Soltys et al. [22] reported the use of a dual-skinned filter membrane allowing convective solute transport in blood to dialysate direction but not in dialysate to blood direction. Finally, membranes with low water permeability but high solute permeability have been created, although these are still just in the experimental stage [20].

Blood and Dialysate Flows

It has been previously observed that backfiltration generally occurs during the first minutes of dialysis, when the blood flow has not yet reached the established regimen [21]. In general, the increase in blood flow represents not only a higher potential clearance for uremic toxins, but also an increase in TMP that could prevent backfiltration. Using high-flux filters, blood flows as high as 500 ml/min have been used without major complications. However, in high water permeability membranes, increasing blood flow might not be enough for maintaining a high TMP along the whole length of the filter. In computer simulations, Yamashita [23] estimated that when increasing blood and dialysate flow to more than 300 and 500 ml/min, respectively, internal filtration can increase from a baseline value of 10 to 40 ml/min. Moreover, the increase of the dialysate flow from 500 to 800 ml/min practically doubles the hydrostatic pressure at the inlet of the dialysate compartment, generating a higher pressure change through the filter which promotes backfiltration [24].

Hematocrit

An increase of hematocrit from 20 to 33% can increase backfiltration from 10 to 15 ml/min/m^2. Of course, at any hematocrit, the increase in the pressure drop associated with higher blood flow rates increases backfiltration further [25].

Fiber Geometry

By maintaining the same total surface area, increasing the inner diameter of the fibers from 200 to 220 μm decreases backfiltration from 15.7 to 11.8 ml/min/m^2. This corresponds to a similar decrement if the length of fibers is shortened from 25 to 21 cm [25]. In this sense, increasing the number of fibers or enlarging their inner diameter while reducing their length would reduce the overall resistance of the filter, producing a reduction of both filtration in its proximal segment and backfiltration in the distal segment [20]. Accordingly, dialysate flow in co-current direction instead of counter-current to blood flow would reduce crossfiltration in general. Of course, all these previously mentioned adjustments would have a negative impact in overall clearance.

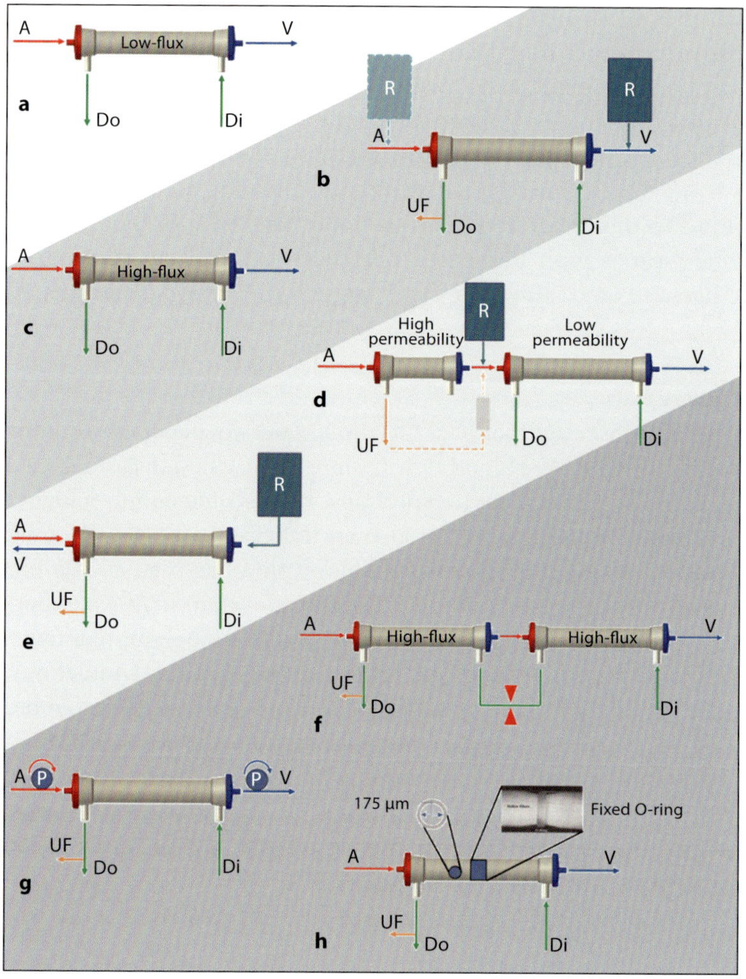

Fig. 2. Different hemodialytic techniques involving backfiltration: (**a**) low-flux HD, (**b**) hemodiafiltration, (**c**) high-flux HD, (**d**) paired filtration dialysis/hemofiltration with reinfusion, (**e**) mid-dilution HDF, (**f**) double high-flux HDF, (**g**) push-pull HDF, and (**h**) enhanced internal filtration HD. White = Minimum backfiltration, Dark gray = maximum backfiltration.

Evolution of Hemodialytic Techniques in Terms of Backfiltration

Low-Flux HD

Backfiltration has a different weighting among the diverse HD techniques (fig. 2). Initially, with low-flux HD, the low water permeability membranes prevented a significant drop in hydrostatic pressure in the blood compartment, maintaining a more constant TMP, less hemoconcentration, and resulted in very low or no probability of backfiltration (although this does not mean no backdiffusion).

High-Flux HD

The introduction of high-flux HD with high water permeability membranes increased the crossfiltration from the blood to the dialysate in the first part of the filter, due to the high TMP obtained by increasing blood flow, and backfiltration in the second part, due to the drop in TMP and hemoconcentration. In contrast to HDF (see below), the UF rate was considerably lower, with an increase in the hydrostatic pressure in the dialysate compartment secondary to the volumetric control by the dialysis machine contributing to backfiltration. This obviously pointed out the erroneous concept that high-flux HD was mostly a diffusive technique.

Hemodiafiltration

The availability of replacement solutions (initially sterile exogenous fluids in a range of 5 to 15 liters per session used in classical HDF and later on-line ultrapure prepared fluids infused at a rate of more than 20 liters per session), allowed an increase of the hydrostatic pressure in the blood compartment and the TMP, promoting more total UF. In the post-dilution modality, a considerable hemoconcentration was generated in the distal part of the filter, favoring backfiltration. Its magnitude again depends upon the water permeability of the membrane. On the other hand, replacement fluid infused in pre-dilution mode could theoretically reduce backfiltration by reducing hemoconcentration inside the hollow fibers [26].

Mid-Dilution HDF

Having mentioned the differences between pre- and post-dilution, a new technique was created to combine both approaches, called mid-dilution HDF. The technique comprises special filters with two longitudinal compartments. The blood passes through the first producing a certain amount of UF. At the end of this, the replacement fluid is added so that hemoconcentration is corrected. Subsequently, blood is redirected to exit in the same entry port. The blood flow in this last section is co-current with the dialysate. The first compartment reproduces post-dilutional HDF and allows backfiltration. Backfiltration is limited in the second, pre-dilutional, compartment. Despite the co-current flow configuration of latter section, high clearances can be obtained due to high convective volumes [26].

Paired Filtration Dialysis and Hemofiltration with Reinfusion

In order to avoid backfiltration, mostly because of concern about water quality, a two-chamber system was conceived by Ghezzi et al. [27] called *paired filtration dialysis*, and was later modified by Ronco et al. [28]. In the first unit, plasma water is removed by UF without the use of dialysate. A sterile replacement solution is reinfused after the first convective filter, and the blood is dialyzed in the second filter equipped with a low-flux low-permeable membrane

[29]. Years later, to avoid an exogenous fluid infusion before the second filter, a new technique called *hemofiltration with reinfusion* was developed in which the ultrafiltrate from the first filter is passed through a sorbent-containing cartridge to retain uremic toxins and then used as replacement fluid. These techniques improve HDF performance by separating the diffusive and convective processes and thus avoiding any interference between them during treatment. Hemofiltration with reinfusion additionally avoids loss of vital molecules during the convective process, such as nutrients, hormones, amino acids or vitamins [29].

Having achieved better standards for water quality, the idea of using backfiltration instead of avoiding it started to be tested. If ultrapure dialysate is employed, substantial amounts of internal filtration and backfiltration could lead to increased convective solute transport across the membrane and to increased dialyzer clearance of middle molecules.

Push-Pull HDF

In push-pull HDF the rotation of a pre-filter blood pump produces filtration (while a post-filter blood pump is stopped), and the rotation of the post-filter pump produces a negative pressure in the blood compartment and thus backfiltration (while the pre-filter pump is stopped). With this system, the blood is concentrated and diluted approximately 25 times before it leaves the hemofilter. It has been reported that up to 120 liters of fluid can be moved in a 4-hour session with high water permeability membranes by this technique [30].

Double High-Flux HDF

In double high-flux HDF, two high-flux dialyzers are placed in series, with the same dialysate flowing through both of them counter-current. By placing a flow restrictor in the dialysate line between the two filters, the first filter which has the arterial port shows a low dialysate pressure favoring filtration. The second filter shows a high dialysate pressure which, together with hemoconcentration, favors fluid substitution by backfiltration under volumetric control. This high efficiency technique was originally created for shortening treatment time down to 2 h per session [31].

Enhanced Internal Filtration HD

Since the beginning of the use of high-flux filters, diverse constructions have been described to enhance the internal filtration in high water-permeable membranes. Yamashita [23] showed that enhancing internal filtration and backfiltration can effectively remove small and middle molecules (cytochrome *c*) in vitro.

Ronco et al. [24] tested a filter modified by a fixed O-ring in the dialysate compartment. This generates a pronounced differential in dialysate pressure, increasing the peaks of positive and negative TMP along the length of the dialyzer. A pronounced drop in the arterial inlet side contributes to filtration, while the increased dialysate pressure in the venous outlet side favors backfiltration. It was estimated that crossfiltration was enhanced by approximately 50% compared to the standard high-flux dialyzer. While clearance for small molecules remained unchanged, inulin and β_2-microglobulin clearances were significantly improved (by 30%).

Applying the Hagen-Poiseuille formula, it is expected that even small changes of the inner diameter of the fiber may result in dramatic changes in its performance [7]:

$$\Delta P = Q_b \times (8\eta l/\pi r^4),$$

where ΔP is the pressure drop along the filter, Q_b is the blood flow, η is the blood viscosity, l is the length of the fiber, and r is the inner radius of the fiber. Dellanna et al. [32] compared β_2-microglobulin removal with 175- and 250-μm diameter fibers. Both had equivalent urea clearance, but a higher flow resistance and TMP produced a higher internal filtration and backfiltration in the filter with the smaller inner diameter, leading to a higher middle molecule removal. In a similar experiment, Ronco et al. [33] compared polysulfone hemodialyzers with fibers of 175 and 200 μm inner diameter. The pressure drop in the blood compartment was higher in the 175-μm fiber dialyzer, leading to an increase in the internal filtration-backfiltration rate from 23.1 to 48.2 ml/min. This resulted in a significant increase of in vivo clearances of vitamin B_{12} and inulin of more than 30%. Moreover, the reduction of the inner diameter increases the average flow velocity per fiber with a consequent increase in wall shear rates; theoretically, this should produce an additional 'cleaning' effect at the blood/membrane interface by reducing the thickness of the protein boundary layer, and therefore improve membrane permeability [7].

Tomo et al. [34] tested a modified 'high fiber density' polysulfone dialyzer as an alternative to enhance internal filtration. At the same time, they improved the structure of the dialyzer housing using a complete surrounding baffle and a slope to allow the uniform diffusion of the dialysate. The results were, again, a clearance of small and middle molecules equivalent to 10 liters of post-dilutional HDF. This equivalence has been confirmed by other authors [33, 35], pointing out the possibility of achieving a good dialytic performance with less complex equipment, no use of replacement solutions, and with an extra barrier for endotoxins and bacteria represented by the polysulfone membrane of the dialyzer itself.

Koda [36] reported a better cost-effectiveness profile for internal filtration-enhanced HD compared to HDF. However, it must be emphasized that loss of proteins, amino acids and water-soluble vitamins can be exacerbated by increasing crossfiltration, so this has to be further evaluated [34, 36].

Conclusions

Backfiltration is a phenomenon that deserves attention as it frequently occurs with the use of high permeability dialysis membranes. First of all, every effort must be made to ensure optimal dialysate and water quality. The availability of ultrapure dialysate has permitted testing of a new paradigm, namely that of using filtration/backfiltration to improve clearance of middle and large molecules. Patient characteristics, dialysis prescription, treatment modality and future modifications in filter and hollow-fiber designs may help us manipulate backfiltration to meet clinical requirements. Backfiltration could become a key factor in performing on-line HDF, with reverse crossfiltration as a mechanism for reinfusion

Acknowledgement

Dr. Vazquez's participation was made possible through the ISN funded Fellowship Program.

References

1 Ronco C, Feriani M, Chiaramonte S, et al: Backfiltration in clinical dialysis. Nature of the phenomenon and possible solutions. Contrib Nephrol. Basel, Karger, 1990, vol 77, pp 96–105.

2 Schmidt M, Baldamus CA, Schoeppe W: Backfiltration in hemodialysis with high permeable membranes. Blood Purif 1984;2: 108–114.

3 Leypoldt JK, Schmidt B, Gurland HJ: Measurement of backfiltration rates during hemodialysis with highly permeable membranes. Blood Purif 1991;9:74–84.

4 Ronco C: Optimization; in Jacobs C, Kjellstrand CM, Koch KM, et al (eds): Replacement of Renal Function by Dialysis, ed 4. Dordrecht, Kluwer Academic, 2004, pp 133–145.

5 Ronco C, Ballestri M, Brendolan A: New developments in hemodialyzers. Blood Purif 2000;18:267–275.

6 Kerr PG, Huang L: Review: membranes for haemodialysis. Nephrology (Carlton) 2010;15:381–385.

7 Ronco C, Brendolan A, Crepaldi C, et al: Flow distribution and cross-filtration in hollow fiber hemodialyzers. Contrib Nephrol. Basel, Karger, 2002, vol 137, pp 120–128.

8 Leunissen KM, Claessens PJ, Mooy JM, et al: Chronic haemodialysis with bicarbonate dialysate. Technical and clinical aspects. Blood Purif 1990;8:347–358.

9 Bland LA, Ridgeway MR, Aguero SM, et al: Potential bacteriologic and endotoxin hazards associated with liquid bicarbonate concentrate. ASAIO Trans 1987;33:542–545.

10 Favero MS, Petersen NJ, Boyer KM, et al: Microbial contamination of renal dialysis systems and associated health risks. Trans Am Soc Artif Intern Organs 1974;20A:175–183.

11 Yamagami S, Adachi T, Sugimura T, et al: Detection of endotoxin antibody in long-term dialysis patients. Int J Artif Organs 1990;13:205–210.

12 Laude-Sharp M, Caroff M, Simard L, et al: Induction of IL-1 during hemodialysis: transmembrane passage of intact endotoxins (LPS). Kidney Int 1990;38:1089–1094.

13 Panichi V, De Pietro S, Andreini B, et al: Cytokine production in haemodiafiltration: a multicentre study. Nephrol Dial Transplant 1998;13:1737–1744.
14 IOS: Quality of dialysis fluid for haemodialysis and related therapies; in ISO 11663. International Organization for Standardization, 2009.
15 Section IV: Dialysis fluid purity. Nephrol Dial Transplant 2002;17(suppl 7):45–62.
16 Schiffl H: High-flux dialyzers, backfiltration, and dialysis fluid quality. Semin Dial 2011;24:1–4.
17 Ronco C, Cappelli G, Ballestri M, et al: On line filtration of dialysate: structural and functional features of an asymmetric polysulfone hollow fiber ultrafilter (Diaclean). Int J Artif Organs 1994;17:515–520.
18 Pegues DA, Oettinger CW, Bland LA, et al: A prospective study of pyrogenic reactions in hemodialysis patients using bicarbonate dialysis fluids filtered to remove bacteria and endotoxin. J Am Soc Nephrol 1992;3:1002–1007.
19 Lonnemann G, Sereni L, Lemke HD, et al: Pyrogen retention by highly permeable synthetic membranes during in vitro dialysis. Artif Organs 2001;25:951–960.
20 Ronco C: Backfiltration: a controversial issue in modern dialysis. Int J Artif Organs 1988;11:69–74.
21 Ronco C: Backfiltration in clinical dialysis: nature of the phenomenon, mechanisms and possible solutions. Int J Artif Organs 1990;13:11–21.
22 Soltys PJ, Zydney A, Leypoldt JK, et al: Potential of dual-skinned, high-flux membranes to reduce backtransport in hemodialysis. Kidney Int 2000;58:818–828.
23 Yamashita AC: New dialysis membrane for removal of middle molecule uremic toxins. Am J Kidney Dis 2001;38(4 suppl 1):S217–S219.
24 Ronco C, Orlandini G, Brendolan A, et al: Enhancement of convective transport by internal filtration in a modified experimental hemodialyzer: technical note. Kidney Int 1998;54:979–985.
25 Robertson BC, Curtin C: Effects of EPO therapy on backfiltration of dialysate in high-flux dialysis. ASAIO Trans 1990;36:M447–M452.
26 Ronco C: Evolution of hemodiafiltration. Contrib Nephrol. Basel, Karger, 2007, vol 158, pp 9–19.
27 Ghezzi PM, Frigato G, Fantini GF, et al: Theoretical model and first clinical results of the paired filtration-dialysis. Life Support Syst 1983;1(suppl 1):271–274.
28 Ronco C, Feriani M, Brendolan A, et al: Paired filtration dialysis: studies on efficiency, flow dynamics and hydraulic properties of the system. Blood Purif 1990;8:126–140.
29 De Francisco AL, Pinera C, Heras M, et al: Hemodiafiltration with on-line endogenous reinfusion. Blood Purif 2000;18:231–236.
30 Shinzato T, Maeda K: Push/pull hemodiafiltration. Contrib Nephrol. Basel, Karger, 2007, vol 158, pp 169–176.
31 von Albertini B: Double high-flux hemodiafiltration. Contrib Nephrol. Basel, Karger, 2007, vol 158, pp 161–168.
32 Dellanna F, Wuepper A, Baldamus CA: Internal filtration – advantage in haemodialysis? Nephrol Dial Transplant 1996; 11(suppl 2):83–86.
33 Ronco C, Brendolan A, Lupi A, et al: Effects of a reduced inner diameter of hollow fibers in hemodialyzers. Kidney Int 2000;58:809–817.
34 Tomo T, Matsuyama M, Nakata T, et al: Effect of high fiber density ratio polysulfone dialyzer on protein removal. Blood Purif 2008;26:347–353.
35 Lucchi L, Fiore GB, Guadagni G, et al: Clinical evaluation of internal hemodiafiltration: a diffusive-convective technique performed with internal filtration enhanced high-flux dialyzers. Int J Artif Organs 2004;27:414–419.
36 Koda Y: Internal filtration-enhanced hemodialysis is a cost-effective treatment in view of solute removal. Blood Purif 2004; 22(suppl 2):36–39.

Dr. Claudio Ronco
Department of Nephrology, San Bortolo Hospital
Viale Rodolfi, 37 36100 Vicenza (Italy)
Tel. +39 444 753650
E-Mail cronco@goldnet.it

Krick G, Ronco C (eds): On-Line Hemodiafiltration: The Journey and the Vision.
Contrib Nephrol. Basel, Karger, 2011, vol 175, pp 46–56

Producing On-Line Ultrapure Dialysis Fluid

Beat von Albertini

Clinique Cecil and Service de Néphrologie et Hypertension, Centre Hospitalier et Universitaire Vaudois, Lausanne, Switzerland

Abstract

The process of on-line generation of ultrapure dialysis fluid is a core prerequisite for the safe execution of modern renal replacement therapies such as on-line hemodiafiltration and high-flux hemodialysis. In these extracorporeal treatments with variable degrees of convection, significant volumes of plasma water are removed and replaced with dialysis fluid, which must occur without causing harm to the patient. Historically, on-line generation of sterile and pyrogen-free physiological substitution fluid by the process of membrane ultrafiltration of fresh dialysis fluid has its origin in hemofiltration, a purely convective therapy. Development of this and later therapies is described in the historical context of a successful effort over decades to overcome the above formidable challenge, which was provided jointly by pioneering clinical investigators and a resourceful dialysis industry.

The process of on-line generation of ultrapure dialysis fluid is a core prerequisite for the safe execution of modern renal replacement therapies such as on-line hemodiafiltration (HDF) and, to a lesser extent, high-flux hemodialysis (HD). Unlike in any other field of medicine, these extracorporeal treatments with variable degrees of convection result in the transfer of up to 1 hectoliter per week of dialysis fluid into blood, which must occur without causing harm to the patient. While absolute safety in this respect cannot be achieved, current systems lessen the probability of patients' exposure to microorganisms and pyrogens by a number of steps to diminish the burden of contamination sequentially, starting with the availability of purified water and ending with membrane ultrafiltration to obtain ultrapure dialysis fluid for use in high-flux HD and, after supplemental

In memory of the late Maurizio Gibertoni and Michael J. Lysaght.

redundant ultrafiltration or filtration of this fluid, for sterile and pyrogen-free infusate for use in on-line HDF and hemofiltration (HF). Based primarily on a validated risk analysis provided by the manufacturer of such systems for the probability of breakthrough of bacteria and pyrogens, certain regulatory authorities have approved on-line HDF for clinical use, with the proviso in Europe that the final user complies with the recommendations for use set by the manufacturer of each of such systems, in particular concerning disinfection measures. International standards exist for minimal requirements and guidelines have been developed for preparation of pure water and ultrapure dialysis fluid [1, 2]. Comprehensive reviews on this subject have been published and are highly recommended to be consulted for the clinician embarking on this therapy [3–5].

That the above challenge could be overcome and worldwide millions per year of routine treatments are now carried out safely, can be considered a success story of an effort which has lasted many years. It was achieved by drawing largely on resources available within the dialysis community itself, provided by pioneering clinical investigators and innovations of a very adaptive dialysis industry. For this historical review, this author has been asked to describe how his personal experience gained in this effort has influenced his clinical practice over the years. It is mechanistic, at times anecdotal, and certainly very incomplete in the recognition of the countless important contributions of others, for which he apologizes. It serves him to commemorate two recently deceased dear friends he has encountered early on this path.

Hemofiltration

Historically, the process of on-line generation of sterile and pyrogen-free fluid by membrane ultrafiltration has its origin in HF, a purely convective therapy. It was introduced in 1967 by Henderson, Besarab, Michaels and Bluemle [6], using a polyelectrolyte/polysulfone flat-sheet membrane with poor diffusive but high hydraulic permeability and a tailored sieving limit of 50,000 daltons for convective solute transport. At the Amicon Corp. Allan Michaels had founded, Ford, Strathmann and Lysaght developed in the following years the phase inversion spinning process to produce from this Diaflo® membrane the hollow-fiber Diafilters®. These were used for HF and in 1977 for the innovative technique of Henderson and Beans [7] for production of sterile pyrogen-free electrolyte solution by ultrafiltration. Interest in HF as an alternative to HD received a substantial boost by the seminal formulation of the square meter – hour hypothesis by Babb, Popovich, Christopher and Scribner [8] in 1971. This hypothesis proposed that the shortfalls of diffusive HD in terms of persistence of uremic toxicity in patients were a consequence of the low dialyzability of so-called middle molecules as compared to that of urea with the then available cellulosic membranes. It was based on two clinical observations: (a) that patients on peritoneal dialysis remained free of uremic neuropathy despite higher average urea and creatinine levels and (b) that uremic neuropathy in patients could be arrested and reversed with increasing the length of each HD. Paradoxically, it was this second element of the hypothesis which later invariably stimulated clinical investigators to shorten treatment time with convective therapies.

Clinical HF as a maintenance therapy for ESRD was pioneered by Quellhorst et al. [9] in Germany since 1972. In 1976, more than a dozen clinical investigators presented their results with HF, obtained with flat-sheet filters provided by Rhône-Poulenc and Sartorius, and commercially available parenteral solutions for substitution. This meeting in Germany was also attended by Benjamin T. Burton, Associate Director of the Artificial Kidney Program of the National Institute of Health, resulting in the announcement in 1977 to sponsor a multicenter controlled study comparing HF with HD. Four groups were awarded a contract in the same year: (1) Henderson, University of California, San Diego, (2) Bosch, von Albertini, Geronemus and Glabman, Mount Sinai Medical Center, New York, (3) Quellhorst, Hann-Münden, and (4) Koch and Baldamus, University Hospital, Frankfurt. As a member of the youngest of these groups (average age 35 years) and probably because of his singular relevant qualification of being of native German tongue, this author was sent to Germany and charged with the responsibility of providing the necessary equipment and substitution fluid for conducting the committed-for clinical HF treatments in the study. Thanks to the introductions provided by Mike Lysaght, he gained access to key clinical investigators and industry. Automated gravimetric cyclers for HF were then purchased and imported from Germany, which in contrast proved impossible for substitution fluid due to regulatory obstacles. Inquiries within the industry in the USA were unsuccessful because of FDA regulations limiting the volume of parenteral solutions to 1-liter glass bottles at the time.

A system was therefore developed in early 1978 for the manufacture of sterile and pyrogen-free substitution fluid in the hospital pharmacy, with the help of Phillip Varghese, our dialysis technician. It was designed to include these five steps: (1) purification of tap water by resin column deionization; (2) distillation with a Barnstead still, resulting in sterile water as the base product; (3) admixture of a regular glucose-free acetate liquid dialysis concentrate in a holding tank; (4) removal of microorganisms and pyrogens from the fluid with ultrafiltration in two serial Amicon Diafilter 40®, identical to Henderson's just introduced technique, in a closed semi-automated circuit with the final filling of 4.5 liters each into empty collapsible PVC bags which had been imported from Germany, and (5) steam sterilization of the sealed bags for 30 min at 230°F (110°C). Incidentally, the greatest difficulty in the 3-month development of the system was related to this step. The exhaust cycle of an available disused autoclave in the hospital had to be modified to prevent rupture of the heated bags during forced cooling. This was achieved with the addition of an automated step of maintenance of a higher holding pressure in the autoclave before and during cooling, provided with a standard air-compressor, purchased at Sears & Roebuck for this purpose. Quality control for each manufactured batch before use included chemical analysis, cultures for bacteria and fungi and testing for pyrogens. The live rabbit injection test specified by the USP was later abandoned when the more sensitive assay with limulus lysate became available.

Close to 60,000 liters of substitution fluid were produced in this fashion and used in the patients (21–32 liters per treatment, 3 times weekly). While sterility was documented throughout, a positive result for endotoxins with the limulus-lysate assay was observed at only one instance in retested fluid associated with a pyrogenic reaction of the patient, for which incidentally the rabbit injection test remained negative. Pyrogenic reactions in the patients were observed initially in about 3% of treatments. They were associated with chills and subsequent fever which, after discontinuation of treatment, would disappear without sequelae overnight. No pyrogenic reactions were observed after a reusable Amicon Diafilter 20® was routinely interposed in the infusate line for redundant final on-line filtration during treatments. For the investigators, this uncertainty represented a very stressful preoccupation throughout the study. Lysaght arranged for an expert evaluation of our system by Dinarello and took the author to a visit of Associates of Cape Cod, where he observed the bleeding of suspended live horseshoe crabs (later released to the sea) for use in a more sensitive limulus-lysate endotoxin assay.

The study was completed in 1980 without occurrence of further adverse events for the patients and resulted in progress made in two areas relevant to HF: (a) efficiency was increased by using higher blood flow rates (500+ ml/min) and the addition of a small volume of predilution (20 ml) to the postdilution mode, preventing membrane fouling for filtration by protein concentration polarization during treatment [10], and (b) guidelines were developed for adequate individualized prescription of weekly total filtration volume, based on kinetic analysis of patients' urea generation [11]. For the investigators, an important lasting effect of the experience gained in the study was twofold: it taught them (a) the necessary respect and caution to aim henceforth for the highest purity of any dialysis fluid in their clinical practice, and (b) as one of its earliest users, that with Henderson's technique of membrane ultrafiltration this could be effectively achieved, provided that it occurred as redundant final step on-line before contact with the patients' blood. The Dialfilters® used for this purpose were considered the 'gold standard' of the time. In reality, they were prone to leak because of at times incompletely achieved sealing of the hollow fibers' exterior to the housing with epoxy resin, preventing reliable testing for integrity at manufacture [H. Göhl, pers. commun.]. Retrospectively, the pyrogenic reactions observed during the study were probably related to the passing of undetected endotoxin from concentrate through leaks in the ultrafilters. That redundant final filtration alleviated this problem, was an early demonstration of the validity of fault safety as a concept in the development of on-line therapies.

The preoccupation with adverse effects in patients was not a lesser one for the clinical investigators in Germany, who had access to commercial parenteral solutions for substitution in HF. A number of severe pyrogenic reactions and sepsis, some with fatal outcome, were observed in these years with positive cultures for water-borne Gram-negative bacteria such as *Enterobacter*, *Pseudomonas* and *Corynebacteria* [12]. Recommendations were then made to altogether discontinue their use or to routinely filtrate the solutions with a reusable hemofilter during treatment [13]. The above preoccupation prompted a research effort on endotoxins and pyrogenic reactions, foremost by Koch's group in Hannover, which resulted in important contributions, such as the formulation of the interleukin-1 hypothesis by Henderson, Dinarello, Koch and Shaldon [14].

On-line HF with on-site batch preparation of substitution fluid was pioneered in 1978 by Shaldon, Mion et al. [15] and was performed with sterile and pyrogen-free infusate resulting from sequential steps of ultrafiltration of reverse osmosis-treated water, batch admixture of dialysate concentrate, redundant on-line ultrafiltration and a later added final filtration with a disposable bacterial filter. No pyrogenic reactions in the patients were observed with this system in 3,000 consecutive treatments (60,000 liters), performed in 13 homes (!) and 3 centers. From 1980 on, these and other investigators used the hollow-fiber Gambro hemofilter FH 202® for the treatments and for on-line substitution generation that Göhl et al. [16] had developed in Hechingen. Made of a physically robust asymmetric polyamide membrane with good filtration and porosity size characteristics, it was routinely pressure tested for integrity at manufacture. Gambro, which quickly became the industrial leader in development of HF, introduced in 1983 the U 7000® polyamide ultrafilter and final disposable U 2000® ultrafilter, specifically designed and validated for effective removal of bacteria and pyrogens, for use in the described 3-step configuration for on-line generation of substitution fluid. Three generations of equipment for HF were developed by Gullberg, Nilson, Bergkvist, et al. in Lund, starting in 1980 with the AK-10 HFM 10® system for gravimetric control of substitution with commercial or on-site batch prepared solutions, followed in 1985 by the GHS-10® system with a proportioning unit for continuous on-line generation of substitution solution under flowmetric control, in 1987 the MPS-10® for bicarbonate-based HD and on-line HF and HDF, in 1993 the AK 100 ULTRA®, with integrated U 8000® and final U 2000® ultrafilters, and in 1996 the more sophisticated AK 200 ULTRA® for on-line therapies. Gambro estimated that from 1981 to the beginning of 1993, more than 1.3 million liters of sterile and pyrogen-free infusate had been generated on-line with their systems and safely used in over 50,000 clinical HF and HDF treatments [17].

By this time, the popularity of HF was already waning. Other than for better vascular stability during treatment and better control of hypertension, the observed clinical results failed to demonstrate a clear superiority over HD. The latter had progressed in the intervening years with the introduction of bicarbonate as buffer, replacing rapidly the ill-tolerated acetate in the dialysis fluid. The real challenge leading to the decline of HF resulted from the outcome of the National Cooperative Dialysis Study in 1983, highlighting the critical importance of urea generation and its quantitatively adequate removal for patient survival, which, to a variable extent, had been neglected by clinical investigators with for this purpose inherently less efficient HF.

Hemodiafiltration

Merging the advantages of HD and HF into one modality was achieved with HDF, an intermittent renal replacement therapy of combined high diffusive and convective solute transport, where the total volume of ultrafiltration exceeds the desired weight loss for the patient and is in part substituted with a physiological solution, for which a system with precise net ultrafiltration (UF) control is indispensable. It was introduced independently in 1977 by three different groups of investigators: Kunitomo, Lowrie et al. [18] in Boston, Ota et al. [19] in Japan, and Leber, Wizemann, Schuetterle et al. [20] in Germany. The first two groups used the Toray flow equalizer and Filtryzer® polymethylmethacrylate (PMMA) hollow-fiber dialyzer, while the Fresenius A 2008 system and Rhône-Poulenc RP6® polyacrylonitrile (PAN) plate dialyzer were used in Germany. Common to all three was a coupled gravimetric system for delivery of sterile normal saline or physiological parenteral solution for substitution. Ota, Leber, and after his tragic death in a car accident, Wizemann used HDF to shorten patients' treatment time to 3 × 3 h/week and less.

Self-generation of substitution for HDF was clinically introduced in 1982 by Usuda, Shinzato et al. [21] in Japan, using a push/pull system for periodic filtration of aliquots of plasma water and backfiltration of dialysis fluid during treatment under volumetric control. Shinzato, Maeda et al. [22] reported clinical use of a serial configuration of two dialyzers with a flow restriction in the blood path for ultrafiltration from blood under flow control and backfiltration of dialysis fluid for substitution under volumetric control. Cheung, Leypolt et al. [23] proposed an in-vitro tested hybrid system in a serial configuration of two hollow-fiber hemofilters for self-generation of substitution by backfiltration of on-line filtered sterile and pyrogen-free dialysis fluid under flow control, but lacked equipment to carry it out clinically.

The experience with high blood flow rates in HF stimulated this author to attempt shortening of treatment time without reducing small and large solute removal of either HD or HF. He had the chance to realize this goal by being invited in 1983 to join the group of Shinaberger, Miller and Gardner in Los Angeles. Having significantly contributed to progress in dialysis since its early days, this group had been involved with HF and HDF and had developed an at the time unique closed-circuit volumetric system, obtained from linking two recuperated Drake-Willock double-piston dialysate proportioning systems, which was capable of performing clinical bicarbonate HD, sequential UF-HD, HF and HDF. It was used in 1983 for performing high-flux HDF in a configuration of two serial high-flux dialyzers for optimal diffusion and a simple flow restriction in the countercurrent dialysate circuit for self-adjusting optimal filtration and simultaneous substitution by backfiltration of sterile and pyrogen-free bicarbonate dialysis fluid, obtained from on-line filtration with an Amicon Diafilter 40® for safety [24]. The treatments were well tolerated and no pyrogenic reactions were observed in the patients. Coupled with high blood and dialysate flow rates, unmatched high rates of diffusive and convective solute removal can be achieved with this modality, which was later re-named double high-flux HDF and has been described again recently [25].

Relevant to the topic of this chapter, it retrospectively appears that the above modality pioneered on-line ultrafiltration of fresh dialysis fluid for ultrapurity for use in any clinical diffusive renal replacement therapy. Putative redundant sequential filtration for sterility and pyrogen removal of substitution fluid for HDF was then achieved by the backfiltration across the dialyzer membrane in the extracorporeal circuit. The hollow-fiber dialyzers used in the treatments, made of cellulose acetate, PMMA and polysulfone, were suitable for this purpose. Incidentally, this was also the first time the new Fresenius Hemoflow F 60® was clinically used in the USA, for which in 1983 the author had to obtain personal import permission by the FDA.

On-line HDF with redundant filtration of dialysis fluid for substitution was introduced in 1985 by Canaud, Polaschegg, Mion et al. [26] with one hemodiafilter in a closed-circuit under volumetric control (Fresenius A 2008 C), where fresh dialysis fluid was diverted with an additional pump for on-line filtration for sterility and pyrogen removal with two serial F 60® dialyzers and infused for substitution in post-dilution mode. This configuration was later modified to include on-line filtration of all fresh dialysis fluid and redundant on-line filtration of infusate with the Diasafe plus® system, which was integrated in 1998 into the mature Fresenius Online plus® system for HDF and HF. Gambro introduced in 2001 an equally mature AK 200 ULTRA S® system with two U 8000S® ultrafilters and final U 2000® filter for on-line HDF and HF. In Japan, Nikkiso developed a single patient dialysis system, containing a single dialysis fluid filter and a single-use final filter for HDF. The majority of on-line HDF therapies in this country are performed with central dialysis fluid delivery systems for reverse osmosis water, dialysis fluid proportioning and on-line ultrafiltration, and final redundant on-line filtration for sterility and pyrogen removal at the individual patient stations.

High-Flux Hemodialysis

This modality for efficient simultaneous small and large solute removal has its origin in 1972 with the development by Rhône-Poulenc of the AN69® PAN flat-sheet membrane and its successful clinical introduction by Funck-Brentano, Man, Granger et al. [27] at the Necker Hospital in Paris. Compared to cellulosic Cuprophan®, it had comparable diffusive, but a tenfold higher hydraulic permeability. To prevent excessive weight loss with the clinical use of this membrane, an apparatus with closed-circuit volumetric control of recirculating countercurrent dialysate was developed, consisting of an air-tight non-compliant 60-liter vat of batch-prepared warmed dialysis fluid and a pump for continuous removal of a preset volume from the circuit into a graduated cylinder. This system was the forerunner of all modern dialysis machines with programmable weight loss for the patient, which incidentally the developers had the foresight to get patented, generating substantial royalties for Rhône-Poulenc for two decades. Consistent with the logic of the square meter-hour hypothesis, the demonstrated 2.2 times higher removal rate for vitamin B_{12} (1,335 daltons) led the clinical investigators to reduce the duration of the patients' dialysis in half, from with Cuprophan® 30 h/week to 15 with AN69®. Despite near doubling of pretreatment levels for urea and creatinine, a marked improvement of their well-being was reported and the astounding observation made that patients with paralyzing neuropathy were able to walk again after 6 months of this therapy [28]. The original apparatus was later modified by Rhône-Poulenc (which later became Hospal) and merged with a proportioning unit into the Rhodial 75 with the Cotral® system, where the recirculating dialysate was in part replenished with fresh dialysis fluid periodically during treatment. Further membrane development resulted in the hollow-fiber high-flux AN69 Nephral ST® dialyzer of today.

A single-pass volumetric flow equalizer with two small fixed volume chambers, each separated by a flexible silicone rubber membrane, for repeated cycled filling of degassed fresh dialysis fluid and withdrawing spent dialysate in a closed circuit, was developed in 1978 by Toray in Japan for clinical use of their hollow-fiber Filtryzer® PMMA dialyzer with high diffusive and hydraulic permeability. In the same year, Fresenius developed independently a very similar system for integration to their 2008 (and all subsequent systems) for precise net UF control. From the standpoint of microbiological purity of the dialysis fluid, the complexity of such hydraulic systems favors the risk of colonization with water-borne Gram-negative bacteria. While the original Rhône-Poulenc apparatus and the first Fresenius A 2008 could be steam sterilized, later models of the system, as most modern machines, offer automated cycles for frequent heat and chemical disinfection for this purpose.

Fresenius introduced in 1983 the Hemoflow F 60® hollow-fiber dialyzer with high diffusive and hydraulic permeability, made of an asymmetric membrane of hydrophobic polysulfone and hydrophilic polyvinylpyrrolidone (PVP) copolymer for enhanced diffusive permeability and biocompatibility. It was developed in collaboration with Strathmann at the Berghof Institute and Klein of Gulf South Institute, and industrially developed by Heilmann et al. at Fresenius in St. Wendel. Gambro introduced in 1989 the Polyflux® hollow-fiber high-flux dialyzer made of an asymmetric polyamide/PVP co-polymer membrane that Göhl et al. had developed. Common to the above two membranes is their wettability, which after contact with water renders them impermeable to air. This is used for the automated procedure of an air-pressure holding test for integrity of each dialyzer or filter at manufacture.

Using the highly permeable Hemoflow F 60® with the closed-circuit volumetric control of the 2008 system, Streicher and Schneider in 1985 demonstrated efficient small and large solute (β_2-microglobulin, 12,500 daltons) removal in clinical high-flux HD. They made the relevant observation, by measurement at zero net UF, of transmembrane pressure gradients in opposite directions at inlet and outlet of the dialyzer in the countercurrent circuit, suggesting occurrence of internal filtration of plasma water into dialysate and simultaneous backfiltration of dialysis fluid into blood across the membrane [29]. Based on his experience with backfiltration in HDF, this author, after rejoining Juan P. Bosch at George Washington University and becoming head of a new dialysis unit in 1986, had, with the expert help of our technician Viroy Barlee, all installed Fresenius 2008 systems of the D, E, H series equipped with a pair of Hemoflow® and later Polyflux® high-flux dialyzers for on-line ultrafiltration of fresh dialysis fluid [30]. These were disinfected with a machine cycle of peracetic acid and heat twice daily and exchanged every 3 months. When becoming available after 1989, they were replaced with the validated Diasafe® polysulfone filter system that Fresenius had developed for this purpose. Starting with reverse-osmosis-treated water, from a loop which was disinfected weekly with formaldehyde, dialysis fluid was obtained with this technique for all treatments in the unit of HD, high-efficiency HD, high-flux HD and double high-flux HDF. No pyrogenic reactions were observed in the patients. Monthly testing with culture and endotoxin assay consistently revealed that the used dialysis fluid met and exceeded current standards for ultrapurity. This is also the case for the author's clinical practice in Lausanne since 1996, where, under the vigilance of Jacky Berger, the purity of water is maintained with a DWA-Nephrosafe® system for night-time twice weekly heat disinfection of the water loop. The Diasafe-plus®-filtered ultrapure dialysis fluid is used for all treatments, performed with single-use Gambro Revaclear® polyarylethersulfone dialyzers, with Fresenius 4008 and 5008 systems for high-flux HD and double high-flux HDF and 5008 systems for on-line HDF in post- and low-flow predilution mode for heparin-free dialysis.

Acknowledgements

The author reports no conflict of interest, but wants to express his gratitude for valuable information and help in the preparation of this chapter, provided by Hermann Göhl at Gambro and Thomas Roy at Fresenius.

References

1 ISO International Standard: Quality of dialysis fluid for haemodialysis and related therapies. ISO 2009;11663:1–15.

2 ERA-EDTA: European best practice guidelines for hemodialysis part I, section IV: Dialysis fluid purity. Nephrol Dial Transplant 2002;17(suppl 7):45–62.

3 Ledebo I: On-line preparation of solutions for dialysis: practical aspects versus safety and regulations. J Am Soc Nephrol 2002;13: S78–S83.

4 Capelli G, Ricardi M, Bonucci D, De Amicis S: Quality of water, dialysate and infusate. Contrib Nephrol. Basel, Karger, 2007, vol 158, pp 80–86.

5 Ward RA: Quality management of dialysis fluid for online convective therapies. Contrib Nephrol. Basel, Karger, 2011, vol 168, pp 78–88.

6 Henderson LW, Besarab A, Michaels A, Bluemle LW: Blood purification by ultrafiltration and fluid replacement (diafiltration). Trans Am Soc Artif Intern Organs 1967;16: 216–222.

7 Henderson LW, Beans E: Successful production of sterile pyrogen-free electrolyte solution by ultrafiltration. Kidney Int 1978;14: 522–525.

8 Babb AL, Popovitch RP, Christopher TG, Scribner BH: The genesis of the square meter-hour hypothesis. Trans Am Soc Artif Intern Org 1971;17:81–91.

9 Quellhorst E, Rieger J, Doht B, Beckmann H, Jacob I, Kraft B, Mietzsch G, Scheler F: Treatment of chronic uremia by an ultrafiltration kidney: first clinical experience. Proc Eur Dial Transplant Assoc 1976;13:314–321.

10 Geronemus R, von Albertini B, Glabman S, Kahn T, Moutoussis G, Bosch JP: High-flux hemofiltration: further reduction in treatment time. Proc Clin Dial Transplant Forum 1979;9:125–127.

11 Bosch JP, von Albertini B, Glabman S: Prescription for hemofiltration. Contrib Nephrol. Basel, Karger, 1982, vol 32, pp 137–145.

12 Frei U, Koch KM: Fever and shock during hemofiltration. Contrib Nephrol. Basel, Karger, 1983, vol 36, pp 117–114.

13 Von Herrath D, Schaefer K, Hüfler M, Pauls A, Koch KM: Complications of hemofiltration. Contrib Nephrol. Basel, Karger, 1982, vol 32, pp 146–153.

14 Henderson LW, Dinarello CA, Koch KM, Shaldon S: Interleukin-1 hypothesis. Blood Purif 1983;1:1.

15 Shaldon S, Beau MC, Deschodt G, Flavier JL, Nilsson L, Ramperez P, Mion C: Three years of experience with on-line preparation of sterile pyrogen-free infusate for haemofiltration. Contrib Nephrol. Basel, Karger, 1982, vol 32, pp 161–164.

16 Göhl H, Konstatin P, Gullberg CA: Hemofiltration membranes. Contrib Nephrol. Basel, Karger, 1982, vol 32, pp 20–30.

17 Sternby J: A decade of experience with on-line hemofiltration/hemodiafiltration. Contrib Nephrol. Basel, Karger, 1994, vol 108, pp 1–11.

18 Kunitomo T, Lowrie EG, Kumazawa S, O'Brien M, Lazarus JM, Gottlieb MN, Merill JP: Controlled ultrafiltration (UF) with hemodialysis (HD): analysis of coupling between convective and diffusive mass transfer in a new HD-UF system. Trans Am Soc Artif Intern Organs 1977;23:234–243.

19 Ota K, Suzuki T, Ozaku Y, Hosino T, Agishi T, Sugino N: Short-time hemodiafiltration using polymethylmethacrylate hemofilter. Trans Am Soc Artif Intern Organs 1978;24:454–457.

20 Leber HW, Wizemann V, Goubeaud G, Rawer P, Schuetterle, D: Simultaneous hemofiltration/hemodialysis: an effective alternative to hemofiltration and conventional hemodialysis in the treatment of uremic patients. Clin Nephrol 1978;9:115–121.

21 Usuda M, Shinzato T, Sezaki R, et al: New simultaneous HF and HD with no infusion fluid. Trans Am Soc Artif Organs 1982;28:24–27.

22 Shinzato T, Sezaki R, Usuda R, Maeda K, Ohbayashi S, Toyota T: Infusion-free hemodiafiltration: simultaneous hemofiltration and dialysis with no need for infusion fluid. Artif Organs 1982;6:453–456.

23 Cheung AC, Kato Y, Leypoldt JK, Henderson LW: Hemodiafiltration using a hybrid membrane system for self-generation of diluting fluid. Trans Am Soc Artif Organs 1982;18: 61–65.
24 Miller JH, von Albertini B, Gardner PW, Shinaberger JH: Technical aspects of high-flux hemodiafiltration for adequate short (under two hours) treatment. Trans Am Soc Artif Organs 1984;30:377–381.
25 von Albertini B: Double high-flux hemodiafiltration. Contrib Nephrol. Basel, Karger, 2007, vol 158, pp 161–168.
26 Canaud B, N'Guyen QV, Lagarde C, Stec F, Polaschegg HD, Mion C: Clinical evaluation of a multipurpose dialysis system adequate for hemodialysis or for postdilution hemofiltration/hemodiafiltration with on-line preparation of substitution fluid from dialysate. Contrib Nephrol. Basel, Karger, 1985, vol 46, pp 184–186.
27 Funck-Brentano JL, Sausse A, Man, NK, Granger A, Rondon-Nucete M, Zingraff J, Jungers P: Une nouvelle méthode d'hémodialyse associant une membrane à haute perméabilité pour les moyennes molécules et un bain de dialyse à circuit fermé. Proc Eur Dial Transplant Assoc 1972;9:55–66.
28 Funck-Brentano J, Nguyen K, Sausse A: Effect of more porous dialysis membranes on neuropathic toxins. Kidney Int 1975;7:S51–S57.
29 Streicher E, Schneider H: The next generation of dialysis membranes – barrier or pathways? Contrib Nephrol. Basel, Karger, 1985, vol 44, pp 127–136.
30 von Albertini B, Barlee V, Bosch JP: Online sterile rinse of reprocessed high-flux dialyzers (abstract). Congr Am Soc Nephrol 1987;94A.

Dr. Beat von Albertini
Centre de Dialyse Cecil, Avenue Ruchonnet 30
CH–1003 Lausanne (Switzerland)
Tel. +41 21 343 01 82
E-Mail Beat.vonalbertini@hirslanden.ch

Krick G, Ronco C (eds): On-Line Hemodiafiltration: The Journey and the Vision.
Contrib Nephrol. Basel, Karger, 2011, vol 175, pp 57–68

Membrane Requirements for High-Flux and Convective Therapies

Sudhir Kumar Bowry

BioSciences, Fresenius Medical Care Deutschland GmbH, Bad Homburg, Germany

Abstract

Worldwide, high-flux dialysis (HF-HD) has now surpassed low-flux dialysis (LF-HD) as the predominant treatment modality, recognition that removal of larger uremic retention solutes is desirable for the treatment of patients with end-stage chronic kidney disease (CKD). An even more advanced form of HF-HD in terms of removal of a broad spectrum of uremic toxins is on-line hemodiafiltration (HDF), involving convective transport mechanisms for solute removal. With the modality reaching considerable technical maturity over the last two decades, on-line HDF is now recognized for its clinical efficiency and effectiveness, versatility and safety. Such has been the success of on-line HDF that, in Europe, more patients are treated with on-line HDF than even peritoneal dialysis. Fabrication of high-flux membranes for convective therapies is more than a matter of simply making the membrane 'more open' or of increasing the membrane pore size which is not the only determinant for achieving higher convection. While convective transport of larger uremic retention solutes primarily demands membranes with high hydraulic permeability and sieving capabilities, the making of a modern dialysis membrane involves several other considerations that culminate in the delivery of an effective and safe therapy. In this communication I outline the essential membrane requirements and principles for solute removal by convection, as well of meeting additional features related to the therapy. The basic principles of the membrane manufacturing processes by which desired membrane morphology is derived for the separation phenomena involved in dialysis are further described. An awareness of this enables one to appreciate that, depending on the individual constituents and variations of the manufacturing processes, fabrication of all high-flux membranes entails achieving a balance between the ideal or desired criteria for blood purification. Dialysis membranes for convective therapies, even from the same base polymer, exhibit significant differences in their morphology and thus in their ability to facilitate convection.

The availability, in 1983, of the Fresenius polysulfone membrane was a landmark not only in the history of Fresenius Medical Care but also of dialysis therapy [1]. At a time when the biocompatibility debate caused considerable uncertainty about the long-term application of cellulose-based membranes, the timely introduction of polysulfone as a versatile dialysis membrane material had an additional impact [2]. It facilitated the revival of more efficient, high-volume treatment modalities that had already been shown to realize better blood cleansing but were limited by the unavailability of appropriate technology, including for membranes [3]. Suitable membranes are a prerequisite for modern high-efficiency dialysis therapy modalities to ensure high blood purification and safety.

Membrane Matters in Hemodialysis

Worldwide, high-flux dialysis (HF-HD) has now surpassed low-flux dialysis (LF-HD) as the predominant treatment modality. This, alone, is recognition that more efficient modes of blood purification are beneficial and desirable for the treatment of patients with end-stage chronic kidney disease (CKD) [4]. With prescription of therapies using high-performance membranes expected to increase further, modern membranes need to meet distinct criteria to ensure maximal efficiency and safety in order to enhance patient outcomes over extended periods. The general criteria that define an ideal dialysis membrane have been described previously [5]. With the advent of more advanced treatment modalities in routine dialysis, the needs of modern dialysis membranes have undergone change in recent years. For these therapies, the following three main requirements – all pertaining to membranes – need to be considered (fig. 1a):

The Need to Balance Removal of Larger Toxins with Prevention of Protein Leakage

Efficient removal of excess water and uremic retention solutes ('uremic toxins') that contribute to the uremic syndrome by affecting multiple systems and organs remains the foremost objective of all dialysis therapies. However, ascertaining in vivo toxicity of a given compound is difficult and controversial [6]. Uremic toxins are a heterogeneous group of substances in terms of their source, biological role or significance, association with other proteins and size [7]. Ever since its conception, dialysis is still essentially based on size exclusion principles, that is, the size of uremic toxins in relation to the mean size of the 'pores' of a membrane determines which substances are retained or are able to traverse the membrane barrier. Many factors and conditions influence the size-based transport of substances from the blood to the dialysate compartment, and vice versa [8]. Knowledge of the size range of substances to be removed from uremic blood is

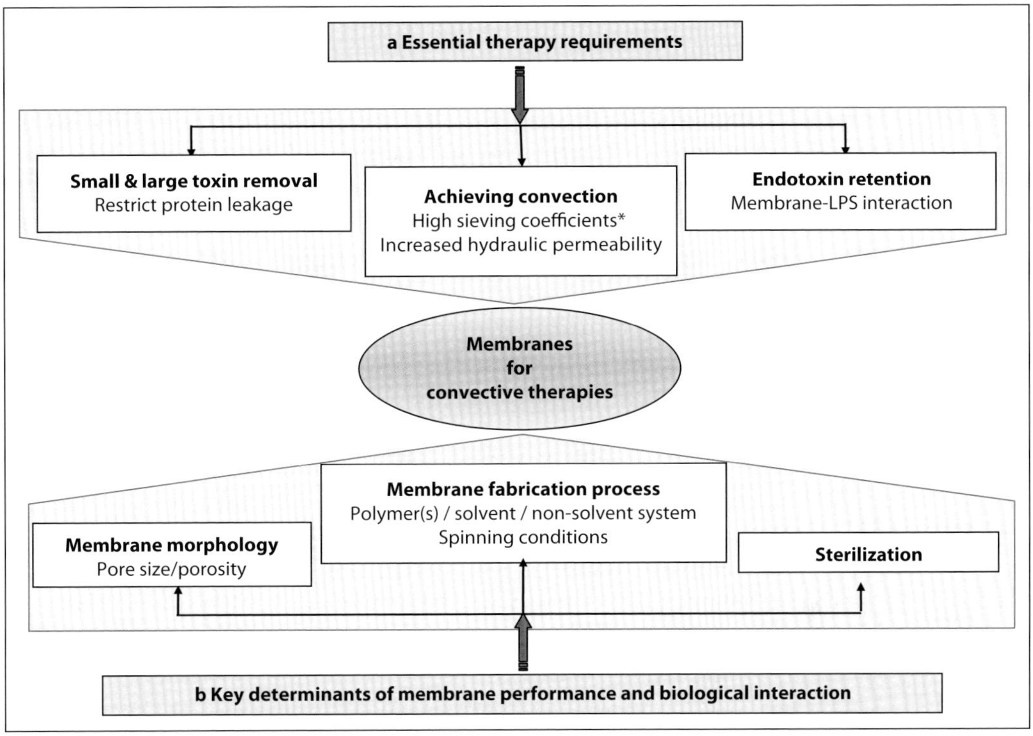

Fig. 1. Essential therapy requirements (**a**) and key determinants of membrane performance and biological interaction (**b**).

thus desirable for the development of appropriate membrane structures. There are other inadvertent mechanisms by which some of the uremic toxin load may additionally be 'removed' during the dialysis. Adsorption of proteins to membrane materials has been well documented and studied, with some membrane materials having a demonstrably higher propensity to overall adsorption of plasma proteins [9]. However, in the opinion and experiences of this author, the phenomenon is highly non-specific, involves virtually all proteins present in blood including those that have little involvement with uremia, varies from one treatment and patient to another and is of minor significance for most dialysis membranes [10]. Furthermore, detecting and quantifying membrane-adsorbed proteins is besieged with methodological difficulties and only monoclonal antibodies are able to identify, or adequately quantify, the constituent proteins of the adsorbed layer.

Considerable advances have been made in recent years in the understanding uremic toxicity. Since its formation in 2000, the European Uremic Toxin (EUTox) Work Group has contributed towards the compilation and classification of an impressive list of substances that are retained in uremia and deemed to be uremic toxins [7, 11]. Newer analytical techniques such as proteomics have enabled an extension of this compilation [12]. Studies examining the kinetics of removal of specific substances reveal the complexity of solute transport from different compartments and aid selection of treatment conditions to facilitate their removal. However, despite such endeavors to ascribe biological significance to individual substances, the extent to which therapeutic strategies have specifically improved or new potential strategies developed as a direct consequence of these deliberations and knowledge is a point of contention. The fact remains that the uremic syndrome can neither be attributed to nor alleviated by removing selected substances, irrespective of how toxic a given substance may be shown to express. The proliferation of studies showing mere associative rather than causal relationships between individual 'uremic toxins' and morbidity-mortality only serves to distract from the non-specific nature of HD therapies. Of the numerous solutes retained and implicated in uremia, only a few (e.g. water, sodium, phosphate, perhaps β_2-microglobulin) could, with a degree of unanimity, be considered uremic 'toxins'. Increased knowledge on uremic toxicity thus reiterates that uremia is attributed to several substances – *small and large* – some perhaps as yet to be identified. In essence, this was advocated when the 'middle molecule hypothesis' was first proposed [13]. With the knowledge we now have and considering how dialysis functions, it is thus more pertinent to consider strategies that remove – as efficiently as possible – the entire size spectrum of uremic toxins regarded as essential to overcoming the effects of uremia and without incurring high albumin loss – rather than consider looking for and targeting specific substances [14]. Difficult as it presently may be, strategies which enable proteins to shed uremic retention solutes bound to them would appear to be much more effective means of achieving enhanced detoxification and improving dialysis therapies [15].

The Need to Achieve More Convection and Larger Exchange Volumes

Once the necessity to eliminate diverse small and large substances is acknowledged, of the available strategies and factors that effect their removal, foremost is the selection of the appropriate treatment modality. Thereafter, other means such as increasing dialysis time (duration) and frequency of treatment as well as selection of treatment conditions such as blood flow according to the individual needs of individual patients are considered to optimize the effectiveness of each treatment session.

Hemodialysis treatment modalities are commonly classified according to membrane 'flux' (from Latin *fluxus, a flowing*, and variant of *fluere, to flow*). The term, together with the prefixes 'low' or 'high' is an indication of the size range of substances a particular membrane or dialyzer is able to remove, i.e. of its relative permeability. As such, low- or high-flux membranes or therapies are highly general terms and do not allude to any specified or defined size ranges of uremic toxins – which themselves are also arbitrarily and variously classified according to solutes being small, middle or large. Such is the generality of the terms 'low flux' and 'high flux' that it is often overlooked that developments in membrane technology, together with product positioning strategies of industry, has led to a change in the meaning and perception of the terms over recent years. Membranes once considered as high flux only a decade or two ago are now categorized as low flux with the consequence that considerable confusion arises during interpretation of published data. In the HEMO Study, for instance, where the effects of flux and dialysis dose on patient survival were examined, dialyzers allocated to the high-flux group can, according to European perspectives, essentially be adjudged as low flux [5].

Patients requiring hemodialysis have the option of the following treatment modalities: LF-HD, HF-HD, HDF (hemodiafiltration) or HF (hemofiltration). Each modality differs in terms of the extent to which it relies on diffusion and convection, the two predominant solute transport mechanisms in dialysis [17]. Adsorption (affinity of molecules for membrane material), as mentioned, is theoretically the third mechanism of removal occurring more by chance than by specific design and cannot precisely be catered for in any of the four treatment options. Thus, the size range (of solutes) as well as magnitude of their removal varies among the four modalities and the treatment conditions selected for each therapy. Diffusive transport, driven by differences in concentrations in the blood and dialysate compartments, has the limitation that the rate of diffusion in free solution decreases with increasing molecular weight [18]. Thus, the relative contribution of diffusion to overall transport decreases the larger the solute. Diffusion also decreases with increasing membrane wall thickness [18]. Convection, which is the predominant mechanism of solute removal across the glomerular membrane, is a consequence of ultrafiltration of fluid across the dialysis membrane wall having a specified structure [17–19]. Ultrafiltration, in turn, is affected by a number of factors such as transmembrane pressure gradient and properties of blood (flow, hematocrit and blood viscosity, plasma proteins, etc.). Both diffusion and convection are determined by the morphological characteristics of the dialysis membrane, i.e. the dimensions (pore size) and structure (degree of porosity) of the membrane wall [8, 20].

To explain diffusion and convection (solute transport) in relation to membrane structure, it is best to conceptualize the membrane wall (mostly 30–40 μm thick) as a dual-layered barrier across which mass transfer is induced: the thin ('skin'), innermost (blood-contacting) region and the bulk 'support' region [21]. The former is also referred to as the separating or sieving region as the dimensions of the pores therein ascertain the size of the substances in the blood that can traverse the membrane and thereby important towards regulation of convective transport. The structure (thickness, degree of porosity or tortuosity) of the latter is important for both diffusion rates and for ultrafiltration [21]. Thus, unlike low-flux membranes, high-flux membranes permit in addition to diffusion, considerably higher convection. An estimate of the contribution of convection to solute transport is most commonly achieved by multiplying the solute sieving coefficient by the ultrafiltration rate [18]:

$$C_{convective} = \text{Sieving coefficient (SC)} \times \text{Ultrafiltration rate (UFR)}$$

The sieving component is determined by the mean pore size at the innermost separating region of the membrane, defining which molecules are retained or are able to traverse the membrane ('cleared'), that is, by the SC for a given molecule [22]. The SC of a specified molecule for a particular membrane is calculated by the solute concentration of the fluid after being filtered by the membrane divided by the difference in the concentration of the solute in fluid (plasma) entering and exiting the dialyzer ($SC = 2\ C_F/C_{Pi} + C_{Po}$). The actual magnitude of convective transport (excluding any effects of adsorption) then depends on how high the UFR rate is, that is, the hydraulic permeability attributed to the support region of the membrane wall [18]. In summary, convection is the extent to which solutes (depending on their sieving at the separating region of the membrane) are 'dragged' along by the removed fluid (depending on hydraulic permeability of the support region of the membrane).

For the four treatment modalities in question, diffusive solute transport decreases in this order: LF-HD ~ HF-HD ~ HDF ~ HF. Solute transport in LF-HD is predominantly based on diffusive principles, having in reality a minor convective component depending on pore dimensions [18]. Conversely, convective transport decreases in this order: HF ~ HDF ~ HF-HD ~ LF-HD, with HF (without fluid in the dialysis compartment) being purely convective, having the highest [18–20]. High-flux membranes are thus used for all modalities except for LF-HD.

Convection and Blood Cleansing: The Significance of Large Exchange Volumes

In convective therapies like HF and HDF, convective transport is maximized by extensive ultrafiltration beyond the volume needed to achieve dry weight [19]. To benefit fully from the convective component for blood purification, large fluid volumes need to be utilized [23]. By operating at peak UFR relative to the blood flow rates achievable for individual patients, high convective clearances for the larger uremic toxins can be achieved [19]. With the availability of large quantities of highly pure dialysis and substitution fluids, prepared 'on-line', UF volumes well beyond 15 liters are commonly realized. Increased convection and removal of large quantities of fluid have been associated with several clinical advantages pertaining to decreased uremic toxin load, anemia correction, reduction of calcium-phosphate product, improved hemodynamic stability and vascular stability and to lower inflammation, an underlying condition of most diseased states. The degree of convective transport is thus decisive from an overall clinical point of view; by removing (and replacing) larger volumes of fluid from the patient during on-line HDF (the most efficient treatment modality removing small and large solutes), more efficient blood cleansing is achieved. Consistent with mechanistic considerations, the results of three independent studies involving large numbers of patients have indicated that a survival advantage is evident with high-volume on-line HDF [24–26]. The volume of substitution, a surrogate of the convective dialysis dose, may thus be considered as a critical factor that may impact patient mortality rates.

The Need to Ensure Safety When Exposing Patients to Large Quantities of Fluids
Typically, at a dialysis fluid flow rate of 500 ml/min, the patient is exposed to some 360 liters of dialysis fluid per week (4 h, 3 times per week), compared to approximately 15 liters/week of fluid intake in individuals with normal renal function. Treatment with on-line HDF may require as many as 25 liters of water per treatment, and if both the frequency and duration of the sessions are increased, the total volume of fluid patients are exposed to is therefore considerable. Thus, the entire production of high-purity dialysis and substitution fluids – from the tap to the patient – involves several steps including water purification systems and special ultrafilters as well as dialyzers with high endotoxin-retention capabilities that ensure chemical and microbiological purity of large volumes of fluid contacting the blood of patients.

Bacterial contamination of dialysis fluids gives rise to endotoxins which have been postulated to adversely impact dialysis outcomes through the stimulation of the inflammatory responses and pathways resulting in oxidative stress. Endotoxins, chemically lipopolysaccharides, are derived from the outer wall of Gram-negative bacteria during cell growth and lysis. During dialysis, they could enter the blood compartment of dialyzers via back-transport (mainly back-filtration) mechanisms. Activation of leukocytes results in the generation of pro-inflammatory cytokines and reactive oxygen species, both of which contribute to cardiovascular disease. Recommendations for the maximum permissible levels of microbiological contamination in terms of bacterial colony-forming units (CFU/ml) and endotoxin units (EU/ml) have been proposed for both water and dialysis fluids. The European Best Practice Guidelines for HD recommends the usage of pure water complying with the standards for all forms and treatment types [27].

Microbiological purity and safety of dialysis fluids is achieved by using special ultrafilters (e.g. DIASAFE® Plus) containing hollow-fiber membranes having a high adsorptive capacity for endotoxins. The endotoxins are retained onto materials such as polysulfone predominantly by the mechanism of hydrophobic-hydrophobic interaction, that is, the hydrophobic part of the endotoxins (the fatty acid chain of the lipid A molecule) binds with the hydrophobic domains of the polysulfone polymer [28]. Ultrapure water is obtained by integrating two such ultrafilters in the dialysis fluid pathway of dialysis machines. The filters can be repeatedly disinfected and used for up to about 100 treatments, or up to a period of 12 weeks. An additional and final line of defense is afforded by certain dialyzers containing hollow-fiber membranes made from synthetic polymers such as polysulfone. A number of studies have shown significant differences between dialysis membranes, even when they are manufactured from the same base polymer, in terms of their safety and ability to prevent passage of endotoxins [22].

The Fabrication of Membranes Meeting the Needs of Modern Convective Therapies

Increasing convection requires membranes having an appropriate structure to enhance removal of larger uremic toxins. Contrary to popular belief and opinion, it is not simply a matter of making the membrane 'more open' or of 'increasing the membrane pore size' which is not the only determinant for achieving higher convection. While convective transport primarily demands high sieving capabilities for larger uremic retention solutes as well as high hydraulic permeability, fabrication of modern membranes involves many other considerations that culminate in the delivery of a safe and effective therapy to the patient (fig. 1b):

Essentials of the Membrane-Making Processes
While one does not need to know how an appliance or a technology is made or functions to be able to use it, an appreciation of the fundamental principles involved nevertheless enables the user to derive maximal benefit from it, or even recognize the limitations. The aforementioned membrane features and functions (e.g. pore size, porosity, sieving ultrafiltration, convection, endotoxin retention, etc.) are frequently and extensively alluded to in the literature, yet rarely in the context of how sophisticated scientific principles and manufacturing conditions transform raw materials into medical devices that replace the functions of a healthy organ.

Fabrication of Membranes by Phase Inversion [29] – The Polymer/Solvent/Non-Solvent Triad
Hollow-fiber membranes are fabricated by the so-called spinning technology similar to the spinning of fibers for textiles. The process involves the controlled transformation of a polymer from a liquid to a solid state. Following selection of the appropriate polymer (or a blend of polymers) for a particular application, the first step is to dissolve the polymer(s) in an appropriate solvent to form a polymer solution. The process of solidification occurs by the transition from one liquid state into two liquids, and at a certain stage during de-mixing the high polymer concentration phase will solidify to form a solid matrix. This is done by injecting the polymer solution through the inner tube of a high-precision spinneret (which determines fiber dimensions) and the emerging fiber is immersed in a coagulation bath containing non-solvent. Here, precipitation occurs as a result of the exchange of solvent with non-solvent which essentially 'extracts'

the solvent from the solution leaving behind a 'scaffolding' structure. By carefully controlling the initial stages of the phase separation processes, the desired membrane morphology for both the innermost separating region (sieving function) and of the support region (ultrafiltration) is derived – according to the desired degree of convection and (target) size range of the uremic toxins that need to be removed.

The Choice of the Polymer System for Convective Membrane Fabrication
The choice of the polymer has, historically, significant implications and connotations regarding the properties it ascribes to the membrane as well as to its impact on the quality or outcome of the therapy. Selection of an appropriate polymer for dialysis membrane manufacture goes beyond the search for alternative polymers instigated by the bioincompatibility of early dialysis membranes made from cellulose, now defunct. The demise of cellulose-based dialysis membranes in the 1980s was further accelerated by the recognition that, unlike cellulose, synthetic materials such as polysulfone were much more versatile in enabling membrane fabrication for convective therapies and removal of middle molecules – both of which were essentially revived because of advancements in technology and a desire to achieve enhanced detoxification [5, 22]. The selection of the polymer begins with its suitability for the phase separation processes that rely on a series of complex thermodynamic principles involving the chemical and physical properties of the spinning solution. Factors such as solution composition, miscibility, homogeneity, viscosity, temperature, humidity, residence time during precipitation, etc., all need to be considered for the selected base polymer. Further, in dialysis where blood compatibility-related issues provoked the search for alternative materials, polymer blends have to be used to attain the hydrophilic-hydrophilic balance for optimal blood-material interactions. Polyvinylpyrrolidone is the most common co-polymer of most modern synthetic dialysis membranes to construe this balance although its usage impacts membrane structure as well [29]. Although chemical and thermal resistance to sterilizing agents (e.g. steam, ethylene oxide and irradiation) are considered at the outset of the polymer(s) selection process, endotoxin-retention capabilities of dialysis membranes are only discernible with the finished product (the dialyzer). Should this crucial prerequisite not be met satisfactorily, the entire membrane-spinning process has to be re-evaluated in terms of revised polymer composition, membrane-spinning conditions, membrane morphology and performance, biocompatibility and endotoxin-retention testing.

Conclusion

Convective therapies are successfully used to treat patients with CKD and acute renal failure [30]. Hemodiafiltration is a treatment modality applied to 14% of

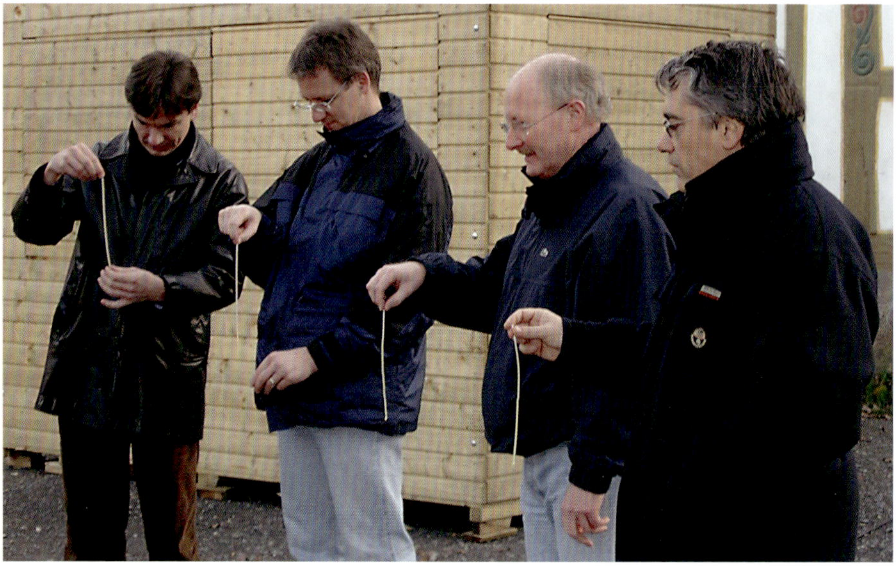

Fig. 2. Leading with verve and skill: Emanuele Gatti has instigated and motivated ideas and innovation to promote OL-HDF by his hands-on approach. Membrane and fibre technology remains a priority under his watchful eye (here demonstrating the art of making wicks from beeswax).

all CKD patients on regular renal replacement therapy in Europe in 2010 and, as such, significantly more patients received HDF than peritoneal dialysis in Europe. Following its conception and early validation, much of the success in the clinical implementation of on-line HDF is to be attributed to technological enterprise, including creating membranes fulfilling functions other than simple sieving demanded by this treatment modality. The contribution and vision of individuals, from scientists and physicians to those in industry, who have steadfastly believed in the virtues of hemodiafiltration for the benefit of the patient, cannot be ignored, and is to be applauded (fig. 2).

References

1 Streicher E, Schneider H: Polysulphone membrane mimicking human glomerular basement membrane. Lancet 1983;322:1136.

2 Brachtendorf T, Nederlof B: Fresenius Polysulfone® – the 'gold standard' in dialysis. Clin Nephrol 1994;42:S3–S12.

3 Henderson LW, Colton CK, Ford CA: Kinetics of hemodiafiltration. II. Clinical characterisation of a new blood cleansing modality. J Clin Lab Med 1975;85:372–391.

4 Koda Y: Clinical outcomes of the high-performance membrane dialyzer. Contrib Nephrol. Basel, Karger, 2011, vol 173, pp 58–69.

5 Bowry SK: Dialysis membranes today. Intern J Artif Organs 2002;25:447–460.
6 Glorieux G, Vanholder R: New uremic toxins – which solutes should be removed? Contrib Nephrol. Basel, Karger, 2011, vol 168, pp 117–128.
7 Vanholder R, De Smet R, Glorieux G, Argilés A, Baurmeister U, Brunet P, Clark W, Cohen G, De Deyn PP, Deppisch R, Descamps-Latscha B, Henle T, Jörres A, Lemke HD, Massy ZA, Passlick-Deetjen J, Rodriguez M, Stegmayr B, Stenvinkel P, Tetta C, Wanner C, Zidek W; European Uremic Toxin Work Group (EUTox). Review on uremic toxins: classification, concentration, and interindividual variability. Kidney Int 2003;63:1934–43.
8 Clark WR, Hamburger RJ, Lysaght MJ: Effect of membrane composition and structure on solute removal and biocompatibility in hemodialysis. Kidney Int 1999;56:2005–2015.
9 Huang Z, Gao D, Letteri JJ, Clark WR: Blood-membrane interactions during dialysis. Semin Dial 2009;22:623–628.
10 Mares J, Thongboonkerd V, Tuma Z, Moravec J, Matejovic M: Specific adsorption of some complement activation proteins to polysulfone dialysis membranes during hemodialysis. Kidney Int 2009;76:404–413.
11 Vanholder R, Argilés A, Baurmeister U, Brunet P, Clark W, Cohen G, De Deyn PP, Deppisch R, Descamps-Latscha B, Henle T, Jorres A, Massy ZA, Rodriguez M, Stegmayr B, Stenvinkel P, Wratten ML: Uremic toxicity: present state of the art. Int J Artif Organs 2001;24:695–725.
12 Weissinger EM, Kaiser T, Meert N, De Smet R, Walden M, Mischak H, Vanholder RC: Proteomics: a novel tool to unravel the patho-physiology of uraemia. Nephrol Dial Transplant 2004;19:3068–3077.
13 Vanholder RC, Glorieux GL, De Smet RV: Back to the future: middle molecules, high-flux membranes and optimal dialysis. Hemodial Int 2003;7:52–57.
14 Krieter DH, Canaud B: High permeability of dialysis membranes: what is the limit of albumin loss? Nephrol Dial Transplant 2003;18:651–654.
15 Watanabe H, Miyamoto Y, Otagiri M, Maruyama T: Update on the pharmacokinetics and redox properties of protein-bound uremic toxins. J Pharm Sci 2011;100:3682–3695.
16 Locatelli F, Gauly A, Czekalski S, Hannedouche T, Jacobson SH, Loureiro A, Martin-Malo A, Papadimitriou M, Passlick-Deetjen J, Ronco C, Vanholder R, Wizemann V; Membrane Permeability Outcome (MPO) Study Group. The MPO Study: just a European HEMO Study or something very different? Blood Purif 2008;26:100–104.
17 Ledebo I: Convective dialysis therapies, current status and perspective. Ther Apher Dial 2005;9:223–227.
18 Ofsthun NJ, Zydney AL: Importance of convection in artificial kidney treatment. Contrib Nephrol. Basel, Karger, 1994, vol 108, pp 53–70.
19 Ledebo I: Principles and practice of hemofiltration and hemodiafiltration. Artif Organs 1998;22:20–25.
20 Ronco C, Ballestri M, Cappelli G: Dialysis membranes in convective treatments. Nephrol Dial Transplant 2000;15:31–36.
21 Ronco C, Bowry S: Nanoscale modulation of the pore dimensions, size distribution and structure of a new polysulfone-based high-flux dialysis membrane. Int J Artif Organs 2001;24:726–735.
22 Bowry S, Gatti E, Vienken J: Contribution of polysulfone membranes to the success of convective dialysis therapies. Contrib Nephrol. Basel, Karger, 2011, vol 173, pp 110–118.
23 Ronco C, Breuer B, Bowry SK: Hemodialysis membranes for high-volume hemodialytic therapies: the application of nanotechnology. Hemodial Int 2006;10:S48–S50.
24 Canaud B, Bragg-Gresham JL, Marshall MR, Desmeules S, Gillespie BW, Depner T, Klassen P, Port FK: Mortality risk for patients receiving hemodiafiltration versus hemodialysis: European results from the DOPPS. Kidney Int 2006;69:2087–2093.
25 Ok E, Asci G, Sevinc-Ok E, Kircelli F, Yilmaz M, Hur E, Sezis M, Demirci M, Ozdogan O, Demirci C, Onen Sertoz O, Duman S, Ozkahya M, Kayikcioglu M, Elbi H, Basci A, Toz H: Comparison of postdilution online hemodiafiltration and hemodialysis (Turkish HDF Study). ERA-EDTA 2011, LBCT2.

26 Grooteman M, Van den Dorpel R, Bots M, Penne L, Van der Weerd N, Mazairac A, den Hoedt CL, van der Tweel I, Lévesque R, Nubé M, Ter Wee P, Blankestijn P: Online hemodiafiltration versus low-flux hemodialysis: effects on all-cause mortality and cardiovascular events in a randomized controlled trial. The Convective Transport Study (CONTRAST). ERA-EDTA 2011, LBCT1.
27 Ward RA: Worldwide guidelines for the preparation and quality management of dialysis fluid and their implementation. Blood Purif 2009;27:2–4.
28 Lonnemann G: Chronic inflammation in hemodialysis: the role of contaminated dialysate. Blood Purif 2000;18:214–223.
29 Mulder M: Basic Principle of Membrane Technology. Dordrecht, Kluwer Academic, 1998.
30 Ronco C, Cruz D: Hemodiafiltration history, technology, and clinical results. Adv Chronic Kidney Dis 2007;14:231–243.

Sudhir Kumar Bowry
BioSciences, Fresenius Medical Care Deutschland GmbH
Else-Kroenerstrasse 1, DE–61352 Bad Homburg (Germany)
Tel. +41 6172 609 2128
E-Mail sudhir.bowry@fmc-ag.com

Krick G, Ronco C (eds): On-Line Hemodiafiltration: The Journey and the Vision.
Contrib Nephrol. Basel, Karger, 2011, vol 175, pp 69–73

Regulatory Challenges of On-Line Hemodiafiltration

D. Pirovano

Pirovano Management SPRL, Brussels, Belgium

Abstract

The launch of on-line hemodiafiltration happened at a very peculiar time from the regulatory standpoint. The directives on medical devices were at their very beginning and the medicinal products regulatory regime was considering, after 30 years of operation of Directive 65/65/EEC, whether it was the case to go for greater harmonization. The success in the introduction of the therapy was strictly linked to the possibility of having the entire system approved for the European market according a single procedure. I had the pleasure to be part of the team, which included Dr. Wolfgang Kümmerle and my old friend Dr. Emanuele Gatti, which succeeded in gathering consensus on the classification of the on-line hemodiafiltration system as a medical device.

Setting the Scene

I had the opportunity to work as a consultant for Fresenius some years ago on the regulatory regime applicable to the new concept of dialysis, developed by Fresenius, known as on-line hemodiafiltration.

The first challenge was to understand the product and its components. The new concept was intended to combine hemodialysis and hemofiltration.

The regulatory problem was mainly whether all the components of the on-line hemodiafiltration machine could or could not fall within the scope of the Medical Devices Directives which were at that time entering the regulatory scenario in Europe.

The major point of uncertainty was linked to the 'revolutionary' production of the electrolyte and of the dialysis solution by the machine itself, not using pre-produced solutions as was the case with the traditional hemodialysis and which were considered as drugs.

The advantage of having all components under the same regulatory regime was evident: the requirements for placing on the market a medical device and a drug are different under almost all aspects, starting from the applicable quality system, to the role of clinical investigations and, not least, the authorities responsible for the evaluation.

In particular at the beginning of the 1990s, the medicinal products regulatory regime was not fully harmonized in spite of the existence of a Community directive since 1965 (Directive 65/65/EEC). The system envisaged national authorizations for drugs, which could then be expanded to other countries through the so-called mutual recognition process. This process was neither easy nor quick and too many national deviations rendered it cumbersome and particularly uncertain and expensive. In those days the Commission was starting to consider the creation of a central agency for the approvals of drugs which saw the light only in 1995 (the European Agency for the Evaluation of Medicinal Products, now called European Medicines Agency), but which had a very limited field of operation.

On the basis of the above and in consideration of the work that the Commission was starting on a harmonized regulatory scheme for medical devices (see below), it was evident that the success of the introduction of hemodiafiltration was heavily dependent on the acceptance from the authorities that all components were classified as medical devices.

The History

At the beginning of the 1990s the European Union was finalizing two directives[1] aiming at harmonizing the placing on the market and the putting into service of a set of products used in healthcare which, from then on, were called 'medical devices' also in Europe[2].

The scope of this initiative was twofold: on one side to harmonize the regulatory requirements which were blossoming among the 12 member states which constituted at that time the 'Communauté Européenne', and on the other to clearly set the boundaries between the Medicinal Products legislation and the Medical Devices legislation.

We were in fact at the eve of one of the most phenomenal industrial developments in a single sector: the medical devices world was finding its way as an

[1] Directive 90/385/EEC on Active Implantable Medical Devices and Directive 93/42/EEC on Medical Devices.

[2] 'Medical device' was already a recognized term in the United States since at least 1976 and in the UK, but across the European Community these products were called several different names, some of which quite fancy (the best: *presidi medico chirurgici* in Italy).

alternative or a complement to the well-established Medicinal Product sector and it was clear to the pioneers that the only way to avoid this sector being 'killed in the cradle' was to favor the European market access of these products with a single system, applicable only once and valid throughout the entire Community and to tailor it to its nature (scientific, technological and from the use standpoint) which is profoundly different from the one of the medicinal products.

It was never the intention to criticize the Medicinal Product regulatory system which was in place in Europe since 1965, but rather highlight that such a system was not, in spite of its stringency, going to ensure safe and effective devices on the market since, for example it did not consider the impact of the skills of the doctors using them, which could count up to 90% of the efficacy of the treatment.

Another concept which was marking the difference between devices and drugs was the iterative nature of innovation which characterizes the device sector as opposed to the drug sector. An implantable pacemaker, in its first shape in the late 1950s, was an ugly box, the size of a pack of cigarettes, weighing 64 g and needed to be recharged every week. The latest versions have the size of two 2-euro coins, weigh a few grams, can be implanted in day hospitals, and last several years. The most recent pacemakers use still the same basic concept of the first ones, but have developed technologically, while in the medicinal products area an innovation is generally considered a molecule which has a new unprecedented target receptor. The need to confirm safety and performance or efficacy of the two products is clear, but the methods to verify them cannot be the same because of their very nature.

This concept was hard to transmit (and apparently it is not easy now either). A number of authorities at that time were reluctant to expand the definition of medical device too much. Their intention was to keep many products under the medicinal products regime which was as said before largely of each member state's pertinence.

The new system was based on the so-called 'new approach'. This legislative technique aimed at setting the fundamental principles to be followed in order to guarantee safety and performance of a product, instead of fixing technical requirements which were difficult to agree on at political level. This was particularly true for the medical devices sector where there are some 400,000 'things' which fall under the definition and are designed and produced by a variety of different types of manufacturers (chemical, mechanical, electrical, electronic, etc.).

Another fundamental characteristic of the new approach was the separation of the duties and responsibilities in the pre- and post-marketing phase. While the evaluation pre-market should have been carried by independent third parties (notified by the National Authorities), the overall surveillance of the market was of pertinence of the various National Competent Authorities.

Finally, it was apparent that not all the 400,000 'things' being medical devices needed the same degree of pre-market third-party evaluation: where the inherent risks related to the use of a tongue depressor could well be minimized under the sole responsibility of the manufacturer, the risk minimization related to the use of a heart valve needed to be verified by a third party before allowing the manufacturer to introduce the device on the market. A risk-based system was then put in place to classify medical devices into 4 classes with a gradual increase of the role of the third-party evaluation depending on the human vulnerability in case of failure of the device.

Those days, I had the honor to be chosen as technical expert within the Directorate General III of the European Commission to advise the Commission services on the technical issues pertinent to devices and I contributed to the drafting and negotiation of the directives.

The challenge was extremely fascinating for me who had been among the very first engineers to graduate from the Politecnico of Milan who were introduced to healthcare engineering. One of the other pioneers of this group of young 'bioengineers' was a certain Emanuele Gatti, with whom I had the chance and the pleasure to work with on different occasions for the last 30 years.

When the contract with the Commission expired and I started my career as a consultant, I was approached by Dr. Gatti who explained to me the challenges that Fresenius was facing in the acceptance from the authorities of the fact that all the components of the on-line hemodiafiltration system had to be considered as a medical device.

I then started working with Dr. Gatti and Dr. Wolfgang Kümmerle, who will surely contribute more technical details than me in another chapter of this book, and together we studied an appropriate rationale for the justification of the classification of on-line hemodiafiltration as a device.

We were lucky enough to find receptive ears among the Member States' experts which were sitting in the Classification and Borderline Working Group of the Commission and good enough to produce a solid rationale which supported the classification of the most 'critical' component of hemodiafiltration as a device on the basis of the letter and the spirit of the newborn directive.

The introduction of on-line hemodiafiltration in the treatment of patients then became a reality.

....

Dr. Dario Pirovano is a consultant for regulatory affairs with Eucomed, the European Medical Technology Industry Federation since 2002. He worked in the European Commission for 4 years, where he contributed to the drafting and negotiating of the 90/385/EEC and 93/42/EEC Directives. He has over 30 years of experience in medical technology as designer and regulatory affairs expert. In 1995 he founded Pirovano Management SPRL, a consulting firm advising manufacturers, Notified Bodies and authorities in regulatory matters relating to medical technology. Dario can be considered the historical memory of the development of medical devices regulation in Europe. He holds a Doctorate in Engineering from the Politecnico di Milano.

D. Pirovano
Pirovano Management SPRL
Avenue de Messidor 306/16, BE–1180 Ukkel (Belgium)
E-Mail Dario.Pirovano@eucomed.org

Krick G, Ronco C (eds): On-Line Hemodiafiltration: The Journey and the Vision.
Contrib Nephrol. Basel, Karger, 2011, vol 175, pp 74–80

Facing Regulatory Challenges of On-Line Hemodiafiltration

Wolfgang Kümmerle

Fresenius Medical Care Deutschland GmbH, Bad Homburg, Germany

Abstract

On-line hemodiafiltration (on-line HDF) is the result of a vision that triggered multifarious changes in very different areas. Driven by the idea to offer better medical treatment for renal patients, technological innovations were developed and established that also constituted new challenges in the field of regulatory affairs. The existing regulations predominantly addressed the quality and safety of those products needed to perform dialysis treatment which were supplied by industrial manufacturers. However, the complexity of treatment system required for the provision of on-line fluids demanded a holistic approach encompassing all components involved. Hence, focus was placed not only on single products, but much more on their interfacing, and the clinical infrastructure, in particular, had to undergo substantial changes. The overall understanding of the interaction between such factors, quite different in their nature, was crucial to overcome the arising regulatory obstacles. This essay describes the evolution of the on-line HDF procedure from the regulatory point of view. A simplified diagram demonstrates the path taken from the former regulatory understanding to the realization of necessary changes. That achievement was only possible through 'management of preview' and consequent promotion of technical and medical innovations as well as regulatory re-evaluations.

Point of Departure

Millions of very efficient and safe applications have demonstrated for many years that the on-line hemodiafiltration (on-line HDF) treatment plays a dominant role in dialysis. This place of value rests measurable advantages for patients suffering from end-stage renal disease. The clinical benefits are attributed to the combination of the physical modes of action of hemodialysis (diffusion) and hemofiltration (convection). By combining the two therapy methods, both the small and the middle-sized molecules can be efficiently removed from the patients' blood.

This specific way of treatment, called hemodiafiltration, is particularly beneficial if large volumes of hemofiltration (HF) solution are available as substitution fluids. Before the availability of the on-line procedure, HDF was performed using single-dose HF solution bags. These substitution bags were produced by pharmaceutical companies, filled into large volume plastic containers with capacities of up to 5 liters, sterilized, stored and transported to the dialysis clinics before being eventually applied by the clinical professionals. Due to complex logistic procedures, unfavorable handling and considerable costs, the provision of larger amounts of HF solution bags was limited. Consequently, the development of the on-line procedure was based upon the idea to prepare the dialysis liquids in situ during the treatment, thereby replacing many of the former logistic steps.

In addition to the technological challenges of on-line production of dialysis fluid, this new concept had to overcome high regulatory hurdles – the industrially manufactured single-dose bags are internationally classified as pharmaceuticals. For this reason, health authorities demand conformance with high quality and safety requirements before granting marketing authorization for finished products. Specific quality criteria primarily relate to the chemical purity and the microbiological safety of the ready-for-use solution (fig. 1).

Historically, solutions for parenteral application were manufactured in hospitals under the responsibility of pharmacists. The produced batches were only allowed to be administered to the patients by physicians after final control and release by these pharmacists in their authorized function. On-line prepared solutions, however, manufactured in the course of the treatment and infused into the patient without interim storage, final quality control and batch release were virgin soil, particularly regarding the regulatory assessment.

In any case, the one-line generated products must at least possess the same quality and safety characteristics as those solutions provided by industry.

An initial regulatory analysis of the major components necessary for preparation of on-line dialysis solutions revealed that a combination of medical devices and pharmaceuticals is required (fig. 2, components 1). As a particular difficulty, so-called 'borderline products' were part of the set of obligatory components.

These 'borderline products' had to be assessed and treated with special focus as they were classified differently by the national health authorities of the member states of the European Union (e.g. handled as pharmaceuticals in Germany but as medical devices in the United Kingdom). Dialysis concentrates were 'borderline products' of particular concern because these are essential raw materials for the production of on-line fluids. Shortly before the dialysis treatment, the concentrates are diluted with water of specified quality by electromedical equipment (the dialysis machine) and thus brought to the individual concentration required for the patient. In hemodialysis, dialysis concentrates are used as raw materials for the preparation of a dialysis solution that flows outside of the

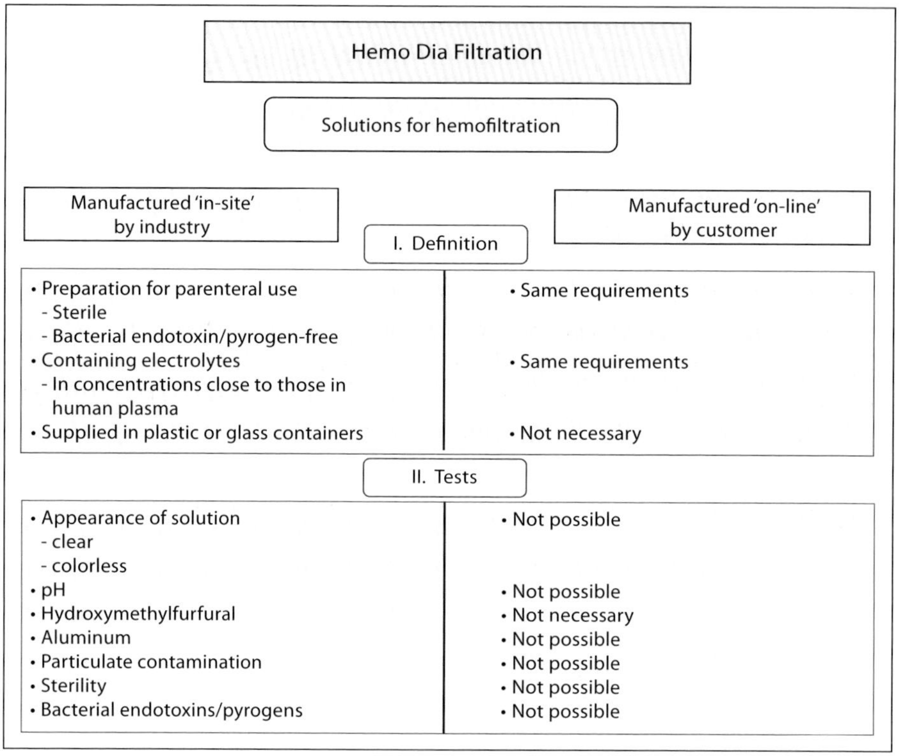

Fig. 1. Quality requirements for HF solutions.

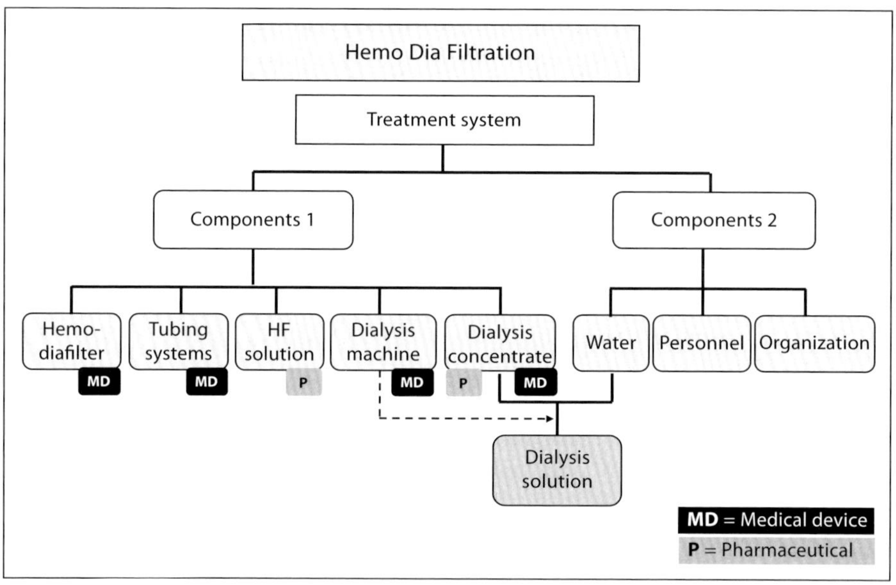

Fig. 2. Essential components for HDF treatment realization.

dialyzer membrane in a direction countercurrent to the blood flow. During this procedure, undesired, toxic metabolites are removed from the blood by means of purely diffusive action.

The on-line HDF procedure uses the same raw materials and applies the same manufacturing method for the preparation of the solutions. However, the resulting fluid not only passes along the outside of the dialyzer's membrane but it is simultaneously infused into the blood circuit of the patient. This new concept of producing dialysis solutions also for the purpose of direct infusion raised new regulatory challenges.

The main tasks to be solved were the provision of the following evidence: (a) evidence that the raw materials used for the preparation of on-line hemodiafiltration solutions possess the required quality; (b) evidence that the manufacturing procedure for on-line dialysis solutions generates products of the required quality; (c) evidence that the infrastructure in the dialysis clinics ensures the required features (see fig. 1, components 2), and (d) evidence that health authorities and notified bodies grant necessary regulatory approvals for all components concerned.

Evolution of the Regulatory Environment

Realization of the various challenges required a circumspect management, both overseeing the whole chain of necessary components and understanding the mutual dependencies and potential risks triggered by the innovative concept. The barriers then in place threatened to prevent the new system from duly gaining market access. In particular, marketing authorizations of certain essential components required by the on-line system were missing. It was Dr. Emanuele Gatti who first addressed the coherence of the medical expectations, the innovative technology and the arising regulatory barriers by a holistic approach. Fresenius Medical Care (FME) employees and external experts were subsequently brought together to identify the basic regulatory obstacles and propose possible solutions. In particular, this FME initiative was supported since 1994 by Dario Pirovano, a technical expert with profound knowledge and experience in European legislation and co-developer of the draft of the new medical device directives. The common project started with the regulatory analysis of the existing directives, laws and standards regarding their scope and applicability to on-line procedures [1, 2]. The primary target was to have existing regulations either reworked or, if necessary, to have suitable new standards elaborated that considered the state of innovation and the expectations of the different stakeholders.

At that time, the European regulatory bodies were about to review the different national requirements aiming at harmonization and classification of medical devices and pharmaceuticals. During this period, borderline issues were

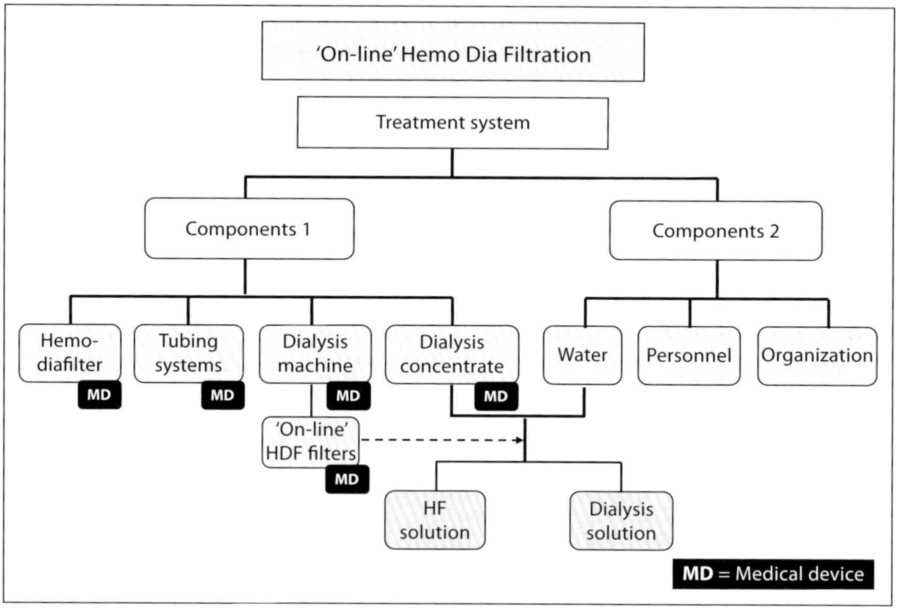

Fig. 3. Essential components for on-line HDF treatment realization.

discussed and assessed by many different parties in order to arrive at a common European understanding. Utmost attention had to be paid to the principal action that the product is intended to perform in or on the patient. After intensive and often controversial discussions of the working group established by the European commission on drug/device borderline issues, the hemodialysis concentrates were allocated to the medical device regulations all over Europe [3]. The explanatory statement concluded that hemodialysis concentrates are medical devices in their own rights as they are '. . .materials . . . used in combination with other medical devices, . . .intended by manufacturers to be used for human beings for the purpose of . . . treating a disease . . . and which do not achieve their principal intended action by pharmacological, immunological or metabolic means' [4]. With this final decision, the pharmaceutical status of concentrates was overcome and all components necessary for the generation of on-line fluids were defined as medical devices in all member states of the European Union and, later on, also beyond the EU borders.

Following this accomplishment, the same regulatory regime could be applied for all components needed for the preparation of on-line in a significant number of target markets. As a consequence, the pharmaceutical regulations had to be replaced by medical device standards and the responsibility switched from the Pharmacopoeia commission bodies to the CEN/CENELEC groups. Without delay, the requirements for the quality of dialysis concentrates were set by a new ISO standard. This norm focused on the hemodialysis procedure and covered 'related therapies', a category that also included innovative on-line procedures [5].

The new international standard mirrors the evolution of European harmonization by stating in the introduction: 'The term consensus . . . does not imply unanimity of opinion, but rather reflects the compromise necessary in some instances when a variety of interests must be merged'. Nevertheless, by the generation of this standard, conscientious efforts of many parties such as physicians, clinical engineers, nurses, dialysis technicians, device manufacturers, notified bodies and governmental representatives succeeded in overcoming regulatory roadblocks for the sake of innovation and, eventually, for the better treatment of dialysis patients.

In the following period, additional ISO standards were established or updated which specified the quality of the water for dialysis and of ready-for-use dialysis fluids [6, 7]. Later, the water preparation equipment was also classified as a medical device in Europe, and the corresponding requirements were specified [8]. FME employees with special expertise steered or participated in the relevant standardization working parties and introduced requirements for on-line HDF treatment. Particular focus was placed on the dialysis machine. This constitutes an essential part of the treatment system because this electromedical device quasi serves as production equipment of the on-line dialysis solution. The development of innovative components and new control mechanisms facilitated the efficient purification of the microbiologically burdened input solution. Double filtration through polysulfone membranes ensured that the resulting output is a sterile, endotoxin-free on-line prepared fluid. Performance, safety and functionality of the on-line HDF equipment were verified by an independent test house. Type testing according to international standards was successfully passed and eventually the CE certification as medical device was granted.

Finally, after all raw materials and system components had gone through the European medical device conformity assessment procedures, all necessary parts for on-line HDF were available for clinical use at full regulatory compliance. Moreover, FME ensured the correct and safe application of the whole treatment system by the definition of rules, procedures and guidelines which were summarized in a dedicated quality management system. FME decided to implement this newly developed clinical quality management system in its company-owned dialysis centers, particularly focusing on the quality and safety of on-line produced fluids. Appropriateness and efficacy of the necessary organization and specified procedures are regularly audited in the FME dialysis centers and assessed by external experts according to internationally recognized standards. The high quality of FME products, clinical infrastructure, medical performance and notably the smooth interplay of all components is virtually demonstrated by the certification according to ISO 9001 standard and Good Dialysis Practice rules.

This integral approach reflects the conviction of the responsible management of FME: quality and safety can be ensured at best if products, personnel and an appropriate infrastructure work together and are continuously improved in a systematic manner by a committed management and motivated personnel.

Conclusion

FME successfully managed the introduction of a complex, multifactorial treatment system which set new standards in dialysis. The innovative approach also triggered changes in the respective regulatory environment in Europe and beyond.

The combined understanding for medical improvement, technological innovation, regulatory evolution, new quality standards and organizational arrangements ensured the realization of a safe and effective therapy system which has been verified to be state-of-the-art in modern dialysis treatment.

It was Dr. Emanuele Gatti who recognized, right from the beginning, the importance of regulatory compliance. He took the lead and oversaw the different aspects involved in the realization of the concept. Besides the identification and motivation of appropriate people for the arising tasks, he brought together diverse disciplines and cultures. This approach resulted in an innovative dialysis therapy system performing safe treatments of high quality which are based upon a new and consistent regulatory regime.

The retrospective assessment of this regulatory evolution concludes an important step from the view of the quality and safety of a single product up to the consideration of the performance of a whole treatment system – a step that is crucial for the meaningful understanding of such a complex therapy system as presented by on-line HDF treatment.

References

1 Pirovano D: Nephrol Dial Transplant 1998;13(suppl 5):21–23.
2 Pirovano D: Regulatory Affairs Focus (3/2000): 31–34.
3 MEDDEV. 14/93 Rev. 4: Guidelines to the Classification of Medical Devices: 8.
4 Council Directive 93/42/42/EEC of June 13 1993 concerning medical devices.
5 ISO 13958: Concentrates for haemodialysis and related therapies.
6 ISO 13959: Water for haemodialysis and related therapies.
7 ISO 11663: Quality of dialysis fluid for haemodialysis and related therapies.
8 ISO 26722: Water treatment equipment for haemodialysis applications and related therapies.

Wolfgang Kümmerle
Fresenius Medical Care Deutschland GmbH
Else-Kröner-Strasse 1, DE–61352 Bad Homburg (Germany)
E-Mail Kuemmerle@fmc-ag.com

Krick G, Ronco C (eds): On-Line Hemodiafiltration: The Journey and the Vision.
Contrib Nephrol. Basel, Karger, 2011, vol 175, pp 81–92

The Membrane Permeability Outcome Study

Francesco Locatelli · Andrea Cavalli · Celestina Manzoni · Giuseppe Pontoriero

Department of Nephrology, Dialysis and Renal Transplant, 'A. Manzoni' Hospital, Lecco, Italy

Abstract

Many observational studies have consistently shown that high-flux hemodialysis has positive effects on the survival and morbidity of uremic patients when compared with low-flux hemodialysis. However, the HEMO study, a randomized trial designed to evaluate the effect of membrane permeability on patient survival, showed only an 8% non-statistically significant reduction of mortality, albeit a secondary analysis suggested an advantage for high-flux membranes in certain patient subgroups. The prospective, randomized Membrane Permeability Outcome (MPO) study investigated the impact of membrane permeability on survival in incident hemodialysis patients who had low albumin (≤4 g/dl) and normal albumin (>4 g/dl) as separate randomization groups. Patients with serum albumin ≤4 g/dl had significantly better survival rates in the high-flux group compared with the low-flux group ($p = 0.032$). Moreover, a post-hoc secondary analysis showed that high-flux membranes may significantly improve survival in diabetic patients. No difference was found in patients with normal albumin levels. Considering the increasing number of dialysis patients with low serum albumin levels and with diabetes, the relevance of the MPO study led to the publication of a position statement by the European Renal Best Practice Advisory Board. This board strongly recommended that high-flux hemodialysis should be used for high-risk patients and, with a lower degree of evidence, even also for low-risk subjects due to the substantial reduction in β_2-microglobulin levels observed in the high-flux group.

The aims of hemodialysis (HD) are to control fluid overload, to correct metabolic acidosis and electrolyte imbalance and to remove the solutes that are normally excreted by the kidneys. However, patient morbidity and mortality rates are still very high today (15–25% per year) [1]. The use of high-flux HD (HF-HD) as an alternative and efficient dialysis technique was proposed more than 20 years ago. It was then believed that the extremely high morbidity and mortality rates were associated with inadequate removal of middle molecular weight solutes and that standard low-flux HD (LF-HD) is not very efficacious in this respect [2]. HF-HD is characterized by the use of membranes of high permeability and increased in vitro clearance of vitamin B_{12} (molecular weight 1,355 daltons), which is considered a marker of middle molecules. Moreover, these membranes remove solutes with molecular weights in excess of that of β_2-microglobulin (11.8 kDa). Good biocompatibility is another key characteristic of high-flux membranes since, during conventional HD with 'bioincompatible' membranes, several cellular mechanisms and biological systems are activated, leading to chronic inflammation and oxidative stress. In uremia, chronic inflammation, together with malnutrition and anemia [3], are considered independent risk factors for accelerated atherosclerosis, cardiovascular complications and death [4]. There are several reasons why chronic inflammation affects uremic patients; here the type of the dialysis membrane and microbial contamination of the dialysate can add to the pro-inflammatory state [5].

What Was the Rationale for the Membrane Permeability Outcome Study?

High-flux membranes are characterized by enhanced removal of middle and high molecular weight solutes that are believed to be involved in the genesis of many complications of HD. After the introduction of HF-HD into clinical practice, several epidemiological and observational studies published since the early 1990s showed an association with an improvement in several aspects of chronic HD-related morbidity. These improvements include a reduction of β_2-microglobulin, a lower incidence of dialysis-related amyloidosis, a slower decrease of residual renal function and a better lipid profile. Furthermore, possible positive effects were also reported for anemia, nutritional status, susceptibility to infection, peripheral nerve conductivity and, above all, long-term survival [6].

Using a data subset from the US Renal Data System (USRDS) registry, Leypoldt et al. [7] showed a clear correlation between death rate and in vitro vitamin B_{12} dialyzer clearance, thus supporting the importance of middle molecules in uremic toxicity. Moreover, recent experimental data has revived interest in middle molecules toxicity [8]. Running parallel to the Membrane Permeability Outcome (MPO) study, the impact of HF-HD on mortality was evaluated in many epidemiologic and observational studies. In an analysis of a sample of the USRDS including nearly 14,000 HD patients, the effect of reuse practice and type of dialyzer membrane were investigated. The results showed that the relative risk for mortality was 24% higher in patients treated with LF-HD than in those receiving HF-HD [9]. A similar reduction (38%) was found in patients on LF-HD versus HF-HD in a European observational cohort of 650 patients [10].

However, no adequately controlled, randomized trials specifically designed to evaluate such benefits have been available for a long time. In 1996, results of a randomized controlled study evaluating the effects of different membrane permeabilities on patient treatment tolerance and nutritional parameters were published [11]. This study did not identify any differences in terms of morbidity or mortality (although it should be underlined that the study was not designed to investigate mortality) [12]. However, this trial was extremely important since it revealed the need to enroll a sicker patient population in future trials in order to adequately address patient mortality. Of note, the conclusions of that study were the basis for the rationale behind the MPO study, which started in 1998.

Thus evidence supporting the clinical superiority of HF-HD was far from being conclusive – there was a clear need for adequate randomized controlled clinical trials to possibly confirm data coming from previous epidemiological studies. For these reasons, two large, randomized and controlled clinical trials were specifically designed to better evaluate the effect of high-flux membranes on morbidity and mortality in HD patients: the Hemodialysis (HEMO) study [12] and the MPO study [13]. The HEMO study, which took place in the United States between 1995 and 2001, evaluated 1,846 mainly prevalent HD patients who were randomized to different membranes and different dialysis doses in a two-by-two factorial design. The aim of the study was to analyze the effect on morbidity and mortality of standard versus high dialysis dose and of low-flux versus high-flux membranes (the latter being defined as having an ultrafiltration coefficient >14 ml/mm Hg per hour) [13]. The trial did not reveal a significant difference in the outcome between the two types of membranes: the adjusted relative risk of all-cause death was with 8% not statistically significantly lower when using high-flux membranes ($p = 0.24$) [13]. A secondary analysis of the study considering only cardiac death or patients receiving HD for more than 3.7 years suggested a better survival in the high-flux group [13]. However, it has to be underlined that the HEMO study, although it is the best trial in the field of dialysis published to date, has some drawbacks, including the following: the relatively low mean age of the patients at inclusion (58 years); the exclusion of patients with low plasma albumin and high body weight; the possible presence of a carry-over effect; the practice of dialyzer reuse, and, above all, the high number of prevalent patients enrolled (selection bias of long survivors). These limitations clearly affect the quality and the general applicability of the HEMO study results [14, 15].

The MPO study was designed to evaluate the long-term effects of membrane permeability on multiple clinical outcomes, including mortality, morbidity, vascular access survival and nutritional status [16]. It is a prospective, randomized, controlled, multicenter clinical trial performed in several European countries. Only incident patients were enrolled (defined as subjects receiving dialysis for no longer than 2 months) to avoid any possible confounding effect of previous treatment schedules and a selection bias towards long survivors [14]. High-flux and low-flux dialyzers were distinguished by their β_2-microglobulin sieving coefficients (>0.6 for HF-HD and 0 for LF-HD) and by their ultrafiltration coefficients (≥20 ml/mm Hg per hour for HF-HD and ≤10 ml/mm Hg per hour for LF-HD). Dialyzer reuse was not allowed [13]. Moreover, the study was specifically designed to include a sicker patient population which, according to the study rationale, is more susceptible to the advantages of HF-HD and in order to provide sufficient statistical power (increased number of events) to possibly demonstrate differences in survival [16]. A serum albumin of ≤4 g/dl was chosen as a marker for increased mortality risk and as an inclusion criterion [16]. However, since the recruitment rate was lower than expected after about 11 months of the enrolment period, and the low albumin requirement was perceived to be the major reason for this, a study amendment was made that also allowed the inclusion of subjects with serum albumin >4 g/dl. A separate randomization list was maintained for these patients to ensure balanced patient distribution and, above all, to facilitate the performance of separate and combined data analysis, thereby avoiding jeopardizing the original study hypothesis.

The trial of Locatelli et al. [11], which provided the basis for the rationale of the MPO study, suggested that dialysis dose is not so relevant for outcome when the dose is higher than a minimum adequate value. Therefore, in order to exclude dialysis dose as a confounding factor in the MPO study, a monitored single pool Kt/V of at least 1.2 was required for patients at randomization and throughout the study. It was thus possible to avoid stratifying the patients and, as a consequence, reducing the statistical power of the study [13]. It is worth noting that the HEMO study was not able to confirm the hypothesis that higher HD dose (Kt/V >1.2) was superior to the standard dose in reducing patient mortality. Thus, the HEMO study proved that CKD-5D patient mortality does not depend on small molecule clearances, provided a threshold minimum dialysis dose is delivered (single pool Kt/V ≈1.3) [12]. Apart from dialysis duration and a minimum dialysis dose, no exclusion criteria were applied in the selection of patients for the MPO study. Thus it was possible to avoid the possibility that the exclusion of high-risk patients could interfere with the results of the study, making the MPO study the first randomized trial evaluating the independent effect of flux on mortality in incident HD patients (table 1).

What Are the Results of the MPO Study?

The MPO study recruitment period lasted 4.5 years, from December 1998 to June 2003, enrolling 738 HD patients from 59 centers in 9 European countries. The number of patients with serum albumin ≤4 g/dl was 567, while 171 patients had serum albumin >4 g/dl. A total of 647 patients were included in the survival analysis (91 subjects could not be considered). Patients in the low-flux and high-flux groups and patients with low and high serum albumin level had similar baseline characteristics [13].

Table 1. Comparison between the HEMO study and the MPO study

	HEMO study	MPO study
Primary outcome	All-cause mortality	All-cause mortality
Study groups and intervention	4 groups 2 × 2 factorial design Membrane flux and dialysis dose	2 groups Membrane flux
Randomization	Stratified by center, diabetic status and age	Stratified by center and serum albumin
Target sample size	900 patients	666 patients
Follow-up	1.5–6.5 years	3–7.5 years
Study sites	USA	9 European countries
Patients	Prevalent patients (≥3 months on HD) Age 18–80 years ≥2.6 g/dl albumin	Incident patients (≤2 months on HD) Age 18–80 years (initially ≤4 g/dl albumin)
Dialyzer	Reuse up to 20 times Synthetic or substituted cellulose	No reuse Synthetic or substituted cellulose (in low-flux group also cellulose)
Results (primary outcome)	Non-statistically significant benefit of high-flux membranes (8% relative risk reduction of mortality)	– Statistically significantly benefit of high-flux membranes for patients with serum albumin ≤4 g/dl (37% relative risk reduction of mortality) – Non-statistically significant benefit of high-flux membranes in the population as a whole (24% relative risk reduction of mortality)
Results (secondary analysis)	Better survival in high-flux group for patients on dialysis for more than 3.7 years or considering cardiac death (22% relative risk reduction)	Better survival in high-flux group for diabetic patients (40.4% relative risk reduction)

Apart from membrane flux, there were no differences between the two groups regarding the dialysis treatment parameters (i.e. blood flow rate, dialysis fluid flow rate, treatment time and dialysis membrane surface area). Membrane flux was clearly different: for patients receiving HF-HD and LF-HD, the mean ultrafiltration coefficient of the dialyzers was 44.7 ± 9.1 and 9.8 ± 3.5 ml/mm Hg per hour, respectively ($p < 0.0001$). The mean dialysis dose was a spKt/V of 1.36 ± 0.3 at month 0 (with no significant difference between the groups);

adjustments to treatment parameters were made during the study course when Kt/V fell below 1.2 or when otherwise indicated [13].

The primary outcome of the MPO study was the effect of membrane permeability on survival in HD patients. This was observed until the last enrolled patient reached 3 years of observation time, until premature termination occurred or until death. The mean study follow-up was 3.0 ± 1.9 years, while the maximum was 7.5 years. During the study, 270 patients prematurely terminated the study: reasons were kidney transplantation, change of dialysis center, withdrawal of patient's consent, change to peritoneal dialysis for >60 days, recovery of renal function or other, not predefined reasons [13].

The initial aim of the study, according to the rationale [11], was to enroll patients at risk. Thus the patients were analyzed separately, according to their serum albumin values. A total of 132 deaths occurred in the group with serum albumin ≤4 g/dl (n = 493) and the crude mortality rate was 8.8%. The difference between the high-flux and the low-flux groups was statistically significant (7.3 vs. 10.4%; p = 0.04). Three- and 4-year mortality rates were 16.9 and 22.3 and 26.6 and 35.7% in the high-flux and the low-flux groups, respectively. A Kaplan-Meier analysis showed that mortality was significantly lower in the high-flux group than in the low-flux group (p = 0.032). The Cox proportional hazards model revealed that membrane permeability reduced the relative risk of mortality by a statistically significant 37% (HR 0.63; 95% CI 0.45–0.90; p = 0.010) [13]. Only 30 patients died in the group with normal serum albumin (>4 g/dl; n = 154). In this set, the 3-year mortality was 19.7% in the high-flux and 16.1% in the low-flux group; the corresponding 4-year mortality was 27.3 and 18.0%, respectively. The survival difference was not statistically significant in the Kaplan-Meier analysis (p = 0.211) [13].

Considering the population as a whole, there were 162 deaths for all causes and a mortality rate of 8.2% during the follow-up of the study; the difference between the two study groups was not statistically significant. Cardiovascular diseases accounted for almost one half of deaths (46.3%), followed by infectious diseases (21.6% of all deaths). The 3-year mortality was 17.0% in the high-flux group and 20.7% in the low-flux group; the corresponding 4-year mortality rates were 26.9 and 31.0%, respectively. Although the Kaplan-Meier analysis showed a slightly better survival in the high-flux group than in the low-flux group, this difference was not statistically significant (p = 0.214). The treatment efficacy analysis revealed comparable results between the two study arms [13]. A Cox proportional hazards model showed that membrane permeability caused a non-statistically significant 24% relative risk reduction of mortality (hazard ratio 0.76; 95% confidence interval 0.56–1.04; p = 0.091). Age, diabetes and comorbidity index were independent predictors of death [13].

Seeing as the number of events is very low in patients with serum albumin >4 g/dl, one can say that the power of the study derives from the initial aim of the trial, which focused only on patients at risk. A secondary post-hoc analysis of survival

Table 2. MPO Study – number needed to treat

	Incidence of events per patient year (×100)		Relative risk reduction	Absolute risk reduction	Number needed to treat
	high-flux	low-flux			
Total patients					
All patients (n = 647)	7.5	9.0	17.3	1.6	63.9
≤4 g/dl albumin (n = 493)	7.3	10.4	30.2	3.2	31.7
Diabetics					
All patients (n = 157)	11.3	18.9	40.4	7.7	13.1
≤4 g/dl Albumin (n = 127)	9.3	20.0	53.3	10.7	9.4

took diabetic patients into consideration (n = 157) and found a higher crude mortality rate in the low-flux group (18.9%) compared to the high-flux group (11.3%): this difference was statistically significant (p = 0.037). In diabetic patients with serum albumin ≤4 g/dl (n = 127), the use of HF-HD resulted in a 53.3% relative risk reduction in mortality and an absolute risk reduction of 10.7% compared to LF-HD (table 2). The Kaplan-Meier survival analysis of diabetic patients as a whole showed a statistically significant higher survival rate in high-flux dialysis compared to low-flux dialysis (p = 0.039). The Cox proportional hazards model (adjusted for age, gender, comorbidity index and vascular access) revealed a 38% relative risk reduction for mortality (hazard ratio 0.62; 95% confidence index 0.38–1.01; p = 0.056) [13]. An interaction was found between the effect of membrane flux and serum albumin levels (p = 0.009) but not with the presence of diabetes (p = 0.216) [13]. This is in contrast to the results of the HEMO study [12].

The MPO secondary outcomes were morbidity and β_2-microglobulin levels. There were no differences in the rate of hospital admissions between the two groups for all causes, for infections or for problems associated to vascular β_2-microglobulin access. β_2-Microglobulin levels were lower in high-flux dialysis than in the low-flux counterpart, with a 3-year increase being statistically significantly different between the study arms (4.4 ± 7.8 vs. 8.0 ± 12.3 mg/l; $p < 0.05$) [13]. These results are of paramount importance considering that the HEMO study reported an association between mortality and β_2-microglobulin levels [17], including mortality for infections [18].

What Is the Clinical Impact of the MPO Study?

In the MPO study, according to the initial study design, high-flux dialysis resulted in a significant lower mortality rate (37% relative risk reduction after adjustment for confounding factors) in patients with serum albumin ≤4 g/dl, i.e. patients considered at risk for poor outcome. However, considering the population as a whole (i.e. including patients with normal and low serum albumin levels), the MPO study did not show a significant effect of membrane permeability on survival [13] – as in the primary analysis of the HEMO study [12]. The authors underlined that the mortality rate of 8.2% is lower than that reported in registries and observational trials, and considered this result to be due to a different patient comorbidity profile (as found in a preliminary study analysis) [19]. It is important to remember that the secondary analysis of HEMO study showed that patients receiving HD for >3.7 years had a relative mortality risk reduction by 32% when treated with HF-HD [12].

The MPO post-hoc analysis, evaluating the effect of membrane permeability in diabetic patients, showed a higher survival rate associated with HF-HD compared to LF-HD, with an adjusted risk reduction of 38%. Although it is important to keep in mind that these results come from a secondary analysis, such data are in line with the rationale of the MPO study [13]. Moreover, a post-hoc analysis of the 4D study [20], which considered only patients receiving HD with the same membrane type during the entire follow-up period, showed that diabetic patients treated with LF-HD had a 59% increase in the hazard ratio for mortality when compared with HF-HD. This further supports the MPO results for diabetic patients.

The MPO study pointed out an interaction of serum albumin with membrane flux. The importance of the results of the MPO study stays in the general applicability of the data found in patients with hypoalbuminemia and diabetes, considering the fact that many dialysis patients have diabetes, inflammation and/or malnutrition [21, 22] (table 2). The causal relation between treatment with HF-HD and improved survival could lie in the eliminative capacity of high-flux membranes, in particular their ability to significantly remove β_2-microglobulin (an acknowledged surrogate of middle molecules) and to reduce its serum levels in the long term, which in turn are related to mortality [17, 18]. Of course, these findings could be related to many factors, including a better volume control as this is more easily achieved with these dialysis techniques (table 3).

The associated editorial comment to MPO study publication by Cheung and Greene [26] underlines the value and insight provided by the MPO study concerning the benefits of HF-HD compared to LF-HD. A key aspect is that the MPO study provided relevant results in a setting that was different from that of the HEMO study. It is noteworthy that, in comparison with the HEMO study, MPO patients were more likely to be white, to use a native fistula and to have less comorbidities. Cheung and Greene [26] pointed out that the fact that subgroup analyses based on serum albumin level were preplanned gives strength to the study findings, reducing possible interferences coming from multiple comparisons. They also suggested that joint analyses of the HEMO and MPO databases should be conducted in order to elucidate any possible combined evidence from

Table 3. Randomized and observational studies evaluating the role of HF-HD on patient mortality

Group (first author)	Design	Treatments	Sample size	Relative risk reduction	p value
Hornberger 1992 [23]	Historical, prospective	HF-HD (107) LF-HD (146)	253	76%	<0.001
Locatelli 1996 [11]	Randomized, prospective	Cuprophan-HD (132) LF-HD (147) HF-HD (51) HDF (50)	380		NS
Koda 1997 [24]	Historical, prospective	HF-HD (248) LF-HD (571)	819	39%	<0.05
Leypoldt 1999 [7]	Historical, prospective	HF-HD LF-HD	1,171	5%	<0.0001
Eknoyan 2006 [12]	Randomized, prospective	HF-HD (921) LF-HD (925)	1,846		NS
Woods, 2000 [25]	Historical, prospective	HF-HD (463) LF-HD (252)	715	42%	<0.01
Port 2001 [9]	Historical, prospective	HF-HD (3,751) LF-HD (9,040)	12,791	19%	0.04
Chauveau 2005 [10]	Historical, prospective	HF-HD (299) LF-HD (351)	650	38%	0.01
Krane 2007 [20]	Post-hoc analysis of prospective randomized study	HF-HD (241) LF-HD (407)	648	59%	0.0006
Locatelli 2009 [13]	Randomized, prospective	Albumin ≤4 g/dl HF-HD (279) LF-HD (283)	562	37%	0.032
	Randomized, prospective	Albumin >4 g/dl HF-HD (84) LF-HD (92)	176		NS
	Randomized, prospective, post-hoc analysis	Diabetics HF-HD (83) LF-HD (74)	157	38%	0.039

the two studies or any new hypotheses that should be tested in new randomized clinical trials. Cheung and Greene [26] finally comment that the results of the MPO study represent the basis for the use of high-flux membranes, with the only limitation being a possible economic burden.

Conclusions

The current European Best Practice Guidelines (EBPG) on dialysis strategies published in 2007 recommend in Guideline 2.1 that 'The use of synthetic high-flux membranes should be considered to delay long-term complications of hemodialysis therapy. Specific indications include: to reduce dialysis-related amyloidosis (evidence level III); to improve control of hyperphosphatemia (level II); to reduce the increased cardiovascular risk (level II), and to improve control of anemia (level III)' [27]. It should be noted that, at the time the guideline was prepared, no sufficient evidence was available to link membrane permeability with survival. The European Renal Best Practice (ERBP) Advisory Board, in the light of the MPO results, recently published a position statement [28] to change the existing Guideline 2.1. The board considered that the MPO study provided sufficient evidence to upgrade the strength of the guidance to a level 1A (strong recommendation, based on high-quality evidence) and recommend that HF-HD should be used in the case of high-risk patients (comparable to the low-albumin group of the MPO study). Because of the substantial improvement in an intermediate marker (β_2-microglobulin) in the high-flux group of the MPO study, the ERBP Advisory Board also recommended that synthetic high-flux membranes should used even in low-risk patients (level 2b: weak recommendation, low quality evidence) [28].

References

1 Cavalli A, Del Vecchio L, Manzoni C, Locatelli F: Hemodialysis: yesterday, today and tomorrow. Minerva Urol Nefrol 2010;62:1–12.

2 Von Albertini B, Miller JH, Gardner PW, Shinaberger JH: High-flux hemodiafiltration: under six hours/week treatment. Trans Am Soc Artif Internal Organs 1984;30:227–231.

3 Carrero JJ, Stenvinkel P: Inflammation in end-stage renal disease- what have we learned in 10 years? Semin Dial 2010;5:498–509.

4 Arici M, Walls J: End-stage renal disease, atherosclerosis, and cardiovascular mortality: is C-reactive protein the missing link? Kidney Int 2001;59:407–414.

5 Himmelfarb J: Uremic toxicity, oxidative stress, and hemodialysis as renal replacement therapy. Semin Dial 2009;22:636–643.

6 Locatelli F, Pozzoni P, Di Filippo S: What are we expecting to learn from the MPO study? Contrib Nephrol. Basel, Karger, 2005, vol 149, pp 83–89.

7 Leypoldt JK, Cheung AK, Carroll CE, Stannard DC, Pereira BJ, Agodoa LY, Port FK: Effect of dialysis membranes and middle molecule removal on chronic hemodialysis patient survival. Am J Kidney Dis 1999;33: 349–355.

8 Vanholder R, Baurmeister U, Brunet P, Cohen G, Glorieux G, Jankowski J, European Uremic Toxin Work Group: A bench to bedside view of uremic toxins. J Am Soc Nephrol 2008;19:863–870.

9 Port FK, Wolfe RA, Hulbert-Shearon TE, Daugirdas JT, Agodoa LY, Jones C, Orzol SM, Held PJ: Mortality risk by hemodialyzer reuse practice and dialyzer membrane characteristics: results from the USRDS dialysis morbidity and mortality study. Am J Kidney Dis 2001;37:276–286.

10 Chauveau P, Nguyen H, Combe C, Chêne G, Azar R, Cano N, Canaud B, Fouque D, Laville M, Leverve X, Roth H, Aparicio M, French Study Group for Nutrition in Dialysis: Dialyzer membrane permeability and survival in hemodialysis patients. Am J Kidney Dis 2005;45:565–571.
11 Locatelli F, Mastrangelo F, Redaelli B, Ronco C, Marcelli D, La Greca G, Orlandini G: Effects of different membranes and dialysis technologies on patient treatment tolerance and nutritional parameters. The Italian Cooperative Dialysis Study Group. Kidney Int 1996;50:1293–1302.
12 Eknoyan G, Beck GJ, Cheung AK, Daugirdas JT, Greene T, Kusek JW, Allon M, Bailey J, Delmez JA, Depner TA, Dwyer JT, Levey AS, Levin NW, Milford E, Ornt DB, Rocco MV, Schulman G, Schwab SJ, Teehan BP, Toto R, Hemodialysis (HEMO) Study Group: Effect of dialysis dose and membrane flux on maintenance hemodialysis. N Engl J Med 2002; 347:2010–2019.
13 Locatelli F, Martin-Malo A, Hannedouche T, Loureiro A, Papadimitriou M, Wizemann V, Jacobson SH, Czekalski S, Ronco C, Vanholder R, Membrane Permeability Outcome (MPO) Study Group: Effect of membrane permeability on survival of hemodialysis patients. J Am Soc Nephrol 2009;20:645–654.
14 Depner TA, Gotch FA, Port FK, Wolfe RA, Lindsay RM, Blake PG, Locatelli F: How will the results of the HEMO study impact dialysis practice? Semin Dial 2003;16:8–21.
15 Locatelli F: Dose of dialysis, convection and haemodialysis patients outcome – what the HEMO study doesn't tell us: the European viewpoint. Nephrol Dial Transplant 2003;18: 1061–1065.
16 Locatelli F, Gauly A, Czekalski S, Hannedouche T, Jacobson SH, Loureiro A, Martin-Malo A, Papadimitriou M, Passlick-Deetjen J, Ronco C, Vanholder R, Wizemann V, for the Membrane Permeability Outcome (MPO) Study Group: The MPO study: just a European HEMO study or something very different? Blood Purif 2008;26:100–104.
17 Cheung AK, Rocco MV, Yan G, Leypoldt JK, Levin NW, Greene T, Agodoa L, Bailey J, Beck GJ, Clark W, Levey AS, Ornt DB, Schulman G, Schwab S, Teehan B, Eknoyan G: Serum β_2-microglobulin levels predict mortality in dialysis patients: Results of the HEMO study. J Am Soc Nephrol 2006;17: 546–555.
18 Cheung AK, Greene T, Leypoldt JK, Yan G, Allon M, Delmez J, Levey AS, Levin NW, Rocco MV, Schulman G, Eknoyan G, HEMO Study Group: Association between serum β_2-microglobulin level and infectious mortality in hemodialysis patients. Clin J Am Soc Nephrol 2008;3:69–77.
19 Locatelli F, Port FK, Pisoni RL, Martin-Malo A, Papadimitriou M, Vanholder R, Hannedouche T, Jacobson SH, Ronco C, Loureiro AC, Wizemann V: Patient and treatment characteristics in the MPO study: validation against the DOPPS population (abstract). Nephrol Dial Transplant 2003; 18(suppl 4):196.
20 Krane V, Krieter DH, Olschewski M, Marz W, Mann JF, Ritz E, Wanner C: Dialyzer membrane characteristics and outcome of patients with type 2 diabetes on maintenance hemodialysis. Am J Kidney Dis 2007;49:267–275.
21 Locatelli F, Manzoni C, Cavalli A, Di Filippo S: Can convective therapies improve dialysis outcomes? Curr Opin Nephrol Hypertens 2009;18:476–480.
22 Locatelli F, Del Vecchio L, Cavalli A: How can prognosis for diabetic ESRD be improved? Semin Dial 2010;23:214–219.
23 Hornberger JC, Chernew M, Petersen J, Garber AM: A multivariate analysis of mortality and hospital admissions with high-flux dialysis. J Am Soc Nephrol 1992;3:1227–1237.
24 Koda Y, Nishi S, Miyazaki S, Haginoshita S, Sakurabayashi T, Suzuki M, Sakai S, Yuasa Y, Hirasawa Y, Nishi T: Switch from conventional to high-flux membrane reduces the risk of carpal tunnel syndrome and mortality of hemodialysis patients. Kidney Int 1997;52: 1096–1101.
25 Woods HF, Nandakumar M: Improved outcome for haemodialysis patients treated with high-flux membranes. Nephrol Dial Transplant 2000;15(suppl 1):36–42.

26 Cheung AK, Greene T: Effect of membrane permeability on survival of hemodialysis patients. J Am Soc Nephrol 2009;20:462–464.
27 Tattersall J, Martin-Malo A, Pedrini L, Basci A, Canaud B, Fouque D, Haage P, Konner K, Kooman J, Pizzarelli F, Tordoir J, Vennegoor M, Wanner C, ter Wee P, Vanholder R: EBPG guideline on dialysis strategies. Nephrol Dial Transplant 2007;22:ii5–ii21.
28 Tattersall J, Canaud B, Heimburger O, Pedrini L, Schneditz D, Van Biesen W, and European Renal Best Practice Advisory Board: High-flux or low-flux dialysis: a position statement following publication of the Membrane Permeability Outcome study. Nephrol Dial Transplant 2010;25:1230–1232.

Prof. Francesco Locatelli
Department of Nephrology, Dialysis and Renal Transplant
Azienda Ospedaliera della Provincia di Lecco, Ospedale 'Alessandro Manzoni'
Via dell'Eremo 9/11, IT–23900 Lecco (Italy)
Tel. +39 0 341 489850, E-Mail f.locatelli@ospedale.lecco.it

Krick G, Ronco C (eds): On-Line Hemodiafiltration: The Journey and the Vision.
Contrib Nephrol. Basel, Karger, 2011, vol 175, pp 93–109

The Early Years of On-Line HDF: How Did It All Start? How Did We Get Here?

Bernard Canaud

Nephrology, Dialysis & Intensive Care Unit, and Institut de Recherche et Formation en Dialyse, Montpellier, France

Abstract

In the mid-1980s, limits and side effects of contemporary hemodialysis were basically due to short treatment time, use of low-flux membranes and employment of acetate-buffered dialysate. These were already associated with a relatively high morbidity and cardiovascular mortality as part of diaysis-related pathology. Based on these considerations, the concept of on-line hemodiafiltration (HDF) was proposed as an innovative solution. By combining diffusive and convective clearances, HDF offered the most efficient modality to clear small and middle-sized uremic toxins. Furthermore, by using ultrapure dialysis fluid and high-flux synthetic membranes, HDF also offered the most biocompatible dialysis system, thereby going a long way towards preventing inflammation. Through provision of virtually unlimited amounts of sterile dialysis fluid by cold sterilization of fresh dialysate, on-line HDF offered an economical and viable method of conducting high-efficiency HDF (high volume exchange) therapy. By keeping the hemodialysis machine with all built-in technical options (e.g. adjustable blood pump, fluid-balancing system, conductivity meter, flow and pressure monitoring, bicarbonate-buffered dialysate), HDF benefited from being associated with the use of dialysis machines with excellent technology as well as highest safety standards. Use of ultrapure water made it then possible to produce dialysis fluid of intravenous grade quality with these machines. The first on-line HDF clinical trial was performed with a modified A2008C dialysis machine in 1984–85. This confirmed the feasibility and potential of the on-line HDF method. Some 25 years later, on-line HDF has proven to be safe, efficacious and with clinical benefits that justify it becoming a new standard for high-quality care of chronic kidney patients.

After three decades of rapid and impressive technical development in renal replacement therapy, dialysis patients were still faced with a high morbidity and mortality risk. Morbidity was reflected in frequent hospitalizations for solving vascular access dysfunction, infection-related problems, cardiovascular events and other dialysis-related pathologies, including β_2-microglobulin amyloidosis. Mortality was high, averaging 17% per year worldwide with large inter-country variations (Japan 7%, Europe 15% and USA 25%). Causes of mortality were predominantly cardiovascular diseases (ischemic cardiac, stroke, arrhythmia, sudden death, etc.) in about 50% of patients, followed by infection, cachexia and various other causes. Several reports identified that, despite multiple adjustments for age, case-mix and comorbidity, the main source of morbidity and mortality in chronic kidney disease patients was the practice of conventional three times weekly, short sessions with low-flux hemodialyzers and acetate-buffered dialysate.

Why Was High-Efficiency Hemodiafiltration Needed in the 1980s to Complete the Armamentarium of Renal Replacement Therapy?

Several hypotheses were proposed to explain the shortfalls in renal replacement therapy. It is not our intention to review the details of the pathophysiological pathways elaborated to elucidate these findings. However, it is important to mention the putative causes and barriers of conventional hemodialysis in order understand the need for designing a more efficient and physiological renal replacement modality. Briefly, the term 'dialysis-related pathology' addresses five main pathophysiological features of the earlier dialysis therapy. First, the incomplete correction of uremic abnormalities by dialysis, this led to the chronic retention of particular toxic compounds [1] and was the focus of attention of the 'uremic toxin group'. In fact, two theories were being followed at that time: the 'small molecule hypothesis' and the 'middle molecule hypothesis'. The 'small molecule hypothesis' was supported by the US nephrology community that uniformly used the 'dialysis dose' concept based on urea Kt/V ratio [2–4]. The 'middle molecule hypothesis', on the other hand, was supported by the European nephrology community that postulated that chronic accumulation of larger molecular size toxins, which are poorly cleared by conventional hemodialysis, were implicated in the high mortality of dialysis patients [5]. The second pathophysiological feature was the 'bioincompatibility' of the hemodialysis system. The generation of bioactive byproducts from protein and cell activation systems led to repetitive inflammation and immune-mediated insults. In this context, two components of the hemodialysis system were identified as triggers for biologic reactions: the biochemical composition of the dialysis membrane (cellulosic versus synthetic polymers) and the microbial contamination of the dialysis fluid [6]. The third pathophysiological aspect of dialysis was the 'hemodynamic instability' of short treatment schedules, accounting for maltolerance in 30–40% of dialysis sessions. Hypotensive episodes induced by dialysis sessions were soon recognized as repetitive cardiac ischemic insults leading, potentially, to myocardial lesions. Apart from high ultrafiltration rate, another factor implicated was the sodium acetate buffering of the dialysate; this was finally proven to play a major role by its vasodilatory and negative inotropic roles in the maltolerance of dialysis sessions [7–9]. The fourth pathophysiological facet was the 'unphysiology' of intermittent therapy that maintained dialysis patients in a permanent unstable situation by creating a 'peak-and-valley' profile of the patient's internal milieu [10]. Finally, the fifth characteristic was the inability to correct 'metabolic abnormalities' of chronic kidney patients, such as anemia, vitamin D deficiency, lipid disorders and mineral and bone disorders [11].

Following reports stressing the limits and side effects associated with short hemodialysis, several technical improvements were proposed for routine clinical practice. This time period led to an intense and fruitful research that contributed to our knowledge and substantially ameliorated outcomes of dialysis patients. In the following, major advances introduced over a short period of time in the dialysis field are briefly reviewed.

Uremic toxins benefited from particular attention. Intense research aimed at their biochemical identification and kinetic characterization, development of specific dosing assays, and proving their toxicity (either in vitro or in animal experiment models) [12]. According to the EUTOX group, uremic toxins are now best classified in three categories based on their molecular size and protein-binding affinity [13]. Although not perfect, this classification has the advantage of underlining difficulties in efficiently clearing middle sized and protein-bound uremic toxins in the clinic setting. As a result, knowledge of uremic toxins is now more comprehensive and strong links to uremic pathology were established. Furthermore, dialyzer manufacturers were prompted to increase membrane permeability and hemodialyzer performances in order to enhance removal of these toxic compounds. Subsequently, high-flux, high-performance, synthetic hemodialyzers (polyacrylnitrile, polysulfone, polyamide, etc.) were developed. Thanks to bioengineering and nanotechnological progress, their performances were optimized. Clinical results were so convincing that their use increased regularly over time so that they are now generally the more prevalent dialzer type worldwide [14–16].

Bicarbonate-buffered dialysate was introduced after the original study from Graefe et al. [17] demonstrated its clear superiority compared to acetate in terms of dialysis tolerance and incidence of hypotensive episodes. Beneficial effects of bicarbonate have been confirmed over time to the point that bicarbonate is nowadays universally the most accepted buffer for dialysate.

Systems for better control of ultrafiltration were developed simultaneously to highly permeable membranes. These systems ensured fluid volume control in dialysis patients during treatment [18]. Beneficial clinical effects were confirmed soon after implementation in hemodialysis machines. This technical option was able to achieve a precise and predictable weight loss associated with a significant improvement in hemodynamic tolerance. Ultrafiltration control systems based on volumetric or flowmetric devices were progressively implemented into the dialysate circuits of all hemodialysis machines, ensuring precise fluid volume balance during highly efficient hemodialysis sessions [19].

Microbiological contamination of water and dialysis fluids was later identified as harmful for dialysis patients. The incidence of fever reactions (pyrogenic reactions) increased significantly after the introduction of bicarbonate-buffered dialysate and high-flux membranes [20]. The link with bicarbonate was soon established and dialysis fluid filtration has since proved to be efficient in preventing fever reactions [21]. More subtly, it was also shown that even low-grade microbial contamination was implicated in monocyte/macrophage activation, resulting in cytokine production and inflammatory reactions [22]. Ultrapurity of water and dialysis fluids was proposed to prevent inflammation and related reactions during hemodialysis sessions [23, 24]. Correcting microinflammation associated with contaminated dialysate is now known to be of paramount importance in preventing the deleterious role of a ubiquitous pathogenic amplifying factor in dialysis patients.

Considering these facts, it became clear to us and others in the mid-1980s that a more effective, gentle and economically viable dialysis modality was required in order to improve outcomes. Ideally, the best suitable treatment modality to achieve this objective had to fulfill several pre-requirements: regular use of highly permeable synthetic membrane hemodialyzers; increased diffusive dialysis dose and maximum convective dose for removal of middle and larger uremic toxins; optimal blood and dialysate flow rates to maximize solute mass transfer; regular use of ultrapure dialysis fluid, and employment of safe and flexible hemodialysis machines capable of mastering balance of fluid volume exchange with multipurpose options for customizing treatment.

Based on these considerations, the concept of on-line hemodiafiltration (HDF) was proposed as an innovative solution. By combining diffusive and convective clearances, HDF offered the most efficient modality to clear small and middle-sized uremic toxins. In vitro and in vivo studies confirmed the superiority of HDF compared to high-flux hemodialysis and high-flux hemofiltration (HF) for removing small and middle-sized uremic toxins [25]. By using ultrapure dialysis fluid and high-flux synthetic membranes, HDF offered in addition the most biocompatible dialysis system. In vitro and in vivo studies showed the beneficial effects in reducing activation of circulating cells and protein systems, and of preventing the induction of inflammation [26]. By providing virtually unlimited amounts of sterile dialysis fluid by cold sterilization of fresh dialysate, on-line HDF offered an economical and viable method to achieve high-efficiency HDF (high volume exchange) therapy. Production of ultrapure dialysis fluid, namely sterile and non-pyrogenic fluid, by ultrafiltration was first reported by Henderson et al. [27, 28] and later successfully applied in a clinic setting, essentially with HF methods. The 'on-line' term was taken from the HF methods that were developed for supply of large volumes of substitution. By keeping the hemodialysis machine with all built-in technology (adjustable blood pump, fluid-balancing system, conductivity meter, flow and pressure monitoring, bicarbonate-buffered dialysate), HDF would rely on the best technical options and most safe dialysis machines.

How Did It All Start?

Discoveries are frequently the fruit of chance and/or personal communications. The birth of on-line HDF may be considered an example of fruitful chance. In the mid-1980s, HF, confusingly named hemodiafiltration by Henderson [29], was presented as the most innovative and promising renal replacement therapy proposed to enhance middle molecule removal and improve chronic kidney disease patient outcomes. Initial clinical studies performed in the USA by Henderson and in Germany by Quellhorst [30, 31] clearly identified the beneficial effects of HF, namely improvement in cardiovascular tolerance and reduction of patient mortality. Due to the gravimetric fluid-balancing system of HF monitors and the bag presentation of substitution electrolyte fluid, the volume of exchange per session was usually limited to 20–25 liters. Low-volume HF appeared insufficient for adequate control of uremia in heavy or non-compliant dialysis patients. In addition, the bag HF method was cumbersome for nurses or technicians, and costly when large volumes of substitution fluid (>40 liters per session) were used. On-line batch preparation was proposed by Shaldon et al. [32, 33] to overcome these difficulties. The feasibility and safety of large volume HF based on on-line batch preparation was assessed in several studies, including a study conducted by our group [34]. Microbiological safety of the batch method was proved in routine clinical practice by applying strict hygiene rules of preparation [35]. Safety of the on-line batch preparation of infusate for HF was also proved using specific HF monitors that included production of ultrapure water from reverse osmosis water [36]. The efficacy of HF with on-line batch substitution fluids was proved to be directly correlated with the substitution volume administered to patient. With the use of on-line batch preparation of substitution fluid, the amount of fluid was no longer limited and the volume of substitution (either in post- or predilutional mode) could be tailored to the metabolic needs of the patient [37]. In order to facilitate the clinical implementation of the batch HF method on a large scale, we developed a central system for producing massive amounts of substitution fluid in closed plastic bags (30 liters). After having overcome the barrier of large volume of infusate, the maximal ultrafiltration rate achievable in clinical practice became the new limiting factor. Despite the use of high blood flow rates (>400 ml/min) and highly permeable hemodialyzers (Kuf >50 ml/mm Hg/h), the mean ultrafiltration rate could not exceed 150 ml/min. This meant that the length of the treatment session needed to be 4–6 h in order to exchange 40–60 liters per session (equivalent to water or urea distribution volume, V) and attain a Kt/V of 1 to 1.2.

Interestingly, during this period, Leber et al. [38] in Germany first reported a new dialysis modality combining diffusive and convective clearances in a high-flux hemodialyzer that they named 'hemodiafiltration'. The term hemodiafiltration, HDF, was well suited to describing the dual action of diffusion (for dialysis) and convection (filtration) occurring within the same filter. In their first clinical experience, the authors underlined the high efficacy and the excellent cardiovascular tolerance of this method. In their original report, which describes the external addition of an infusion pump into the hemodialysis monitor, the sterile electrolyte substitution fluid was delivered in plastic bags (5 liters) and fluid balance was ensured by a gravimetric balancing system that continuously adjusted the ultrafiltration rate to the infusion rate by means of an ultrafiltration pump and a fluid-balancing system in the dialysis machine.

While looking for a more efficient and user-friendly dialysis machine, we were approached by Fresenius to evaluate their new 2008 hemodialysis machine. The A2008C HD machine delivering bicarbonate-buffered dialysate, equipped with a volumetric fluid-balancing module and providing all technical options, was ideally designed to perform HDF. Based on our long experience of producing ultrapure dialysate and infusate, we decided to adapt the 2008 machine to produce on-line substitution fluid. In cooperation with the research and development department of Fresenius and with the help of highly specialized engineers, the 2008 machine was modified: a cold sterilizing ultrafilter was placed in the fresh dialysate circuit ensuring delivery of ultrapure dialysis fluid, an additional infusion module was implemented on the 2008 HD machine consisting of an adjustable infusion pump, and a second sterilizing ultrafilter was placed in the infusate line. The fluid diverted from the fresh dialysate by the infusion pump and infused in the blood drip chamber was isovolumetrically compensated by the ultrafiltrate taken from the patient's blood by the ultrafiltration pump and the fluid-balancing module of the A2008C dialysis machine. A scheme of this original hydraulic circuit modification is given in figure 1. On-line production of substitution fluid from fresh dialysate was born and immediately applied in the clinical treatment of chronic kidney disease patients. The original picture of on-line HDF 2008 machine is presented in figure 2. The first feasibility and safety clinical trial was performed in Montpellier with 4 patients over a 6-week period and reported at the Bad Homburg meeting in 1985 [39]. After this initial trial, the on-line HDF method was progressively expanded to all dialysis patients in our dialysis facilities [40]. Several technical improvements performed on the HDF monitors (2008, 4008 and 5008 series) clearly contributed to geographical spreading of the method. These facilitated clinical handling, enhanced safety, optimized performances by introducing new options for quantifying such, improved cardiovascular tolerance, and developments in substitution

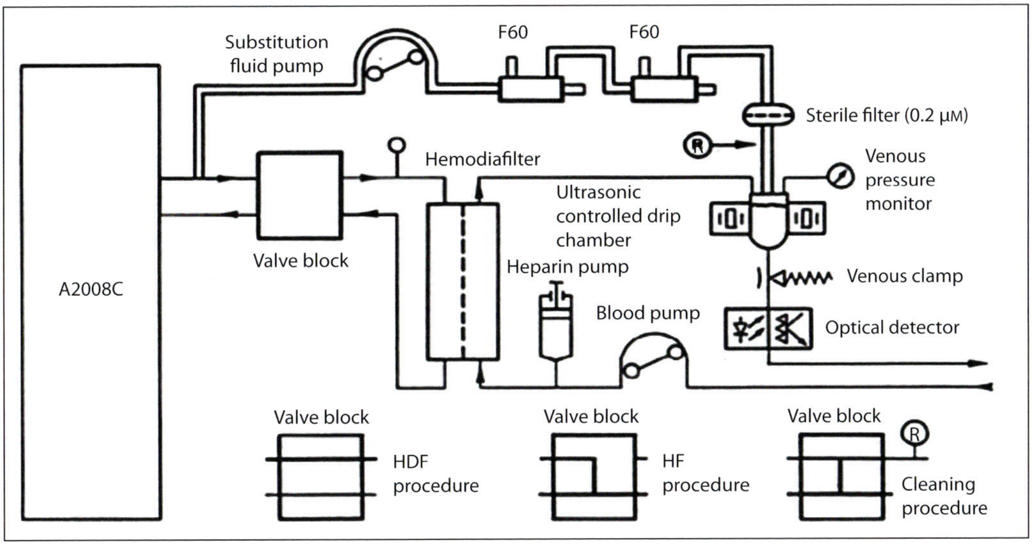

Fig. 1. Modifications of the hydraulic circuit of the A2008C HD machine to perform online HDF as originally done.

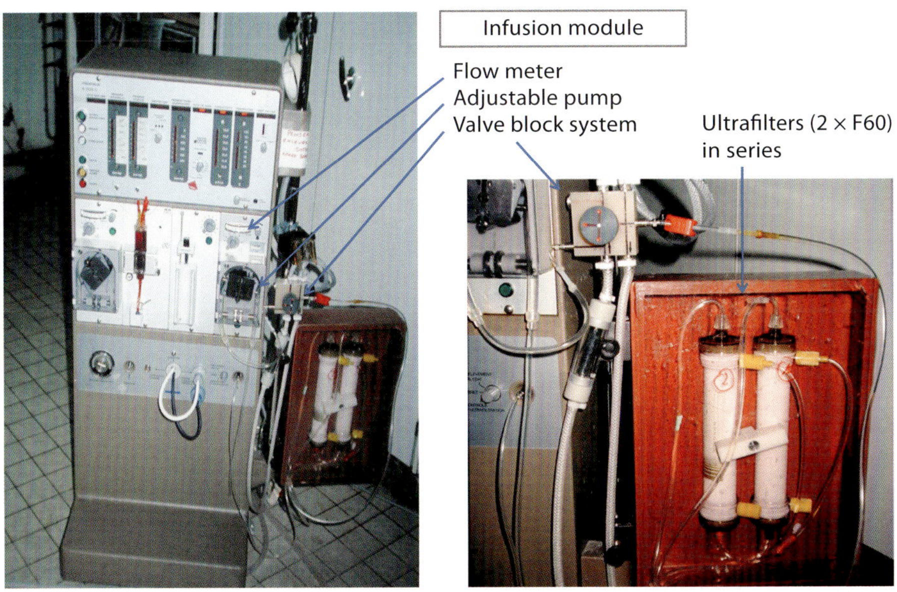

Fig. 2. A2008C HDF machine with its online infusion module and side-kick ultrafilters system.

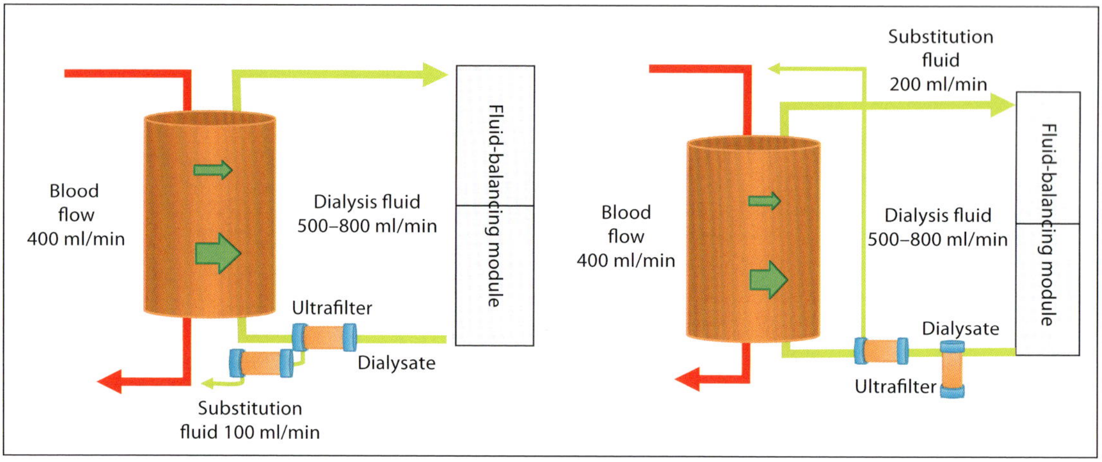

Fig. 3. Configurations of online HDF machines to perform post- or pre-dilution modalities.

possibilities (fig. 3). The evolution of the on-line HDF machines is presented in figures 4 and 5.

How Did We Get Here?

Over the last three decades, on-line HDF has gained in popularity. Such an increase in prevalent use (now more than 1 million HDF sessions have been performed worldwide) has largely confirmed the safety, efficiency and reliability of the method.

On-line production of substitution fluid based on cold sterilization processing of fresh dialysate by ultrafiltration has been proven efficient and safe both in experimental and clinical conditions [41]. Safety and reliability of on-line HDF machines has also been largely proven in routine clinical use over long-term periods, provided the purity of the water feeding into the HD machine is ensured and best clinical practices of hygiene are followed [42]. In addition, on-line techniques have proven to be the only economically viable model, giving access to unlimited amounts of sterile non-pyrogenic fluid [43]. Based on this concept, several alternatives to the post-dilution modality were proposed for optimizing performances of HDF, e.g. pre-dilution HDF, mixed dilution (combined pre- and post-dilution) HDF, or mid-dilution HDF. Interestingly, these options were mainly developed to match the volume of substitution to the metabolic needs of the patient, taking into account the hemorheological changes induced by high hematocrit levels. High hematocrit levels can result from use of erythropoietic-stimulating agents as well as from

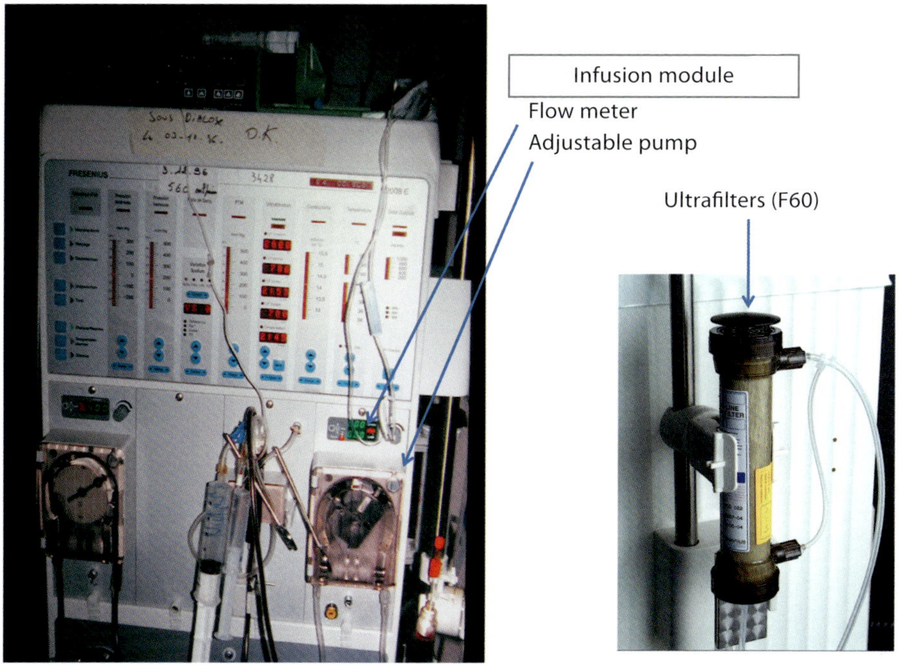

Fig. 4. Evolution of the online HDF machine with the 2008E series.

the phenomenon of hemoconcentration (increase protein concentration) following ultrafiltration.

Best practice guidelines have also been developed to ensure the quality of on-line HDF methods. Best practices incorporate basic hygienic rules of maintenance and disinfection for water treatment systems, fluid distribution systems and the HDF machines themselves in order to prevent microbial contamination and biofilm formation, also within the hydraulic tubings of the machines [44]. This regulation has been reinforced in some specific countries where the on-line methods were particularly applied. A specific working group (EUDIAL) has recently been created within the ERA-EDTA to evaluate and give preferentiality to safe development of on-line methods.

Over the last decade, tremendous technical progress has been made in HDF machines by manufacturers. This ensures safety, reliability and high performance, while simultaneously adding new options to quantify efficacy and to increase the tolerance of sessions. On-line HDF machines now benefit from a specific certification and CE marking by regulatory bodies in the European Community (EC) [45]. This official recognition of CE marking for on-line methods was a major advance in the field of renal replacement therapy. Indeed, it is the first time that a medical device was approved and certified for intravenous infusion of a sterile and non-pyrogenic pharmaceutical product prior to any

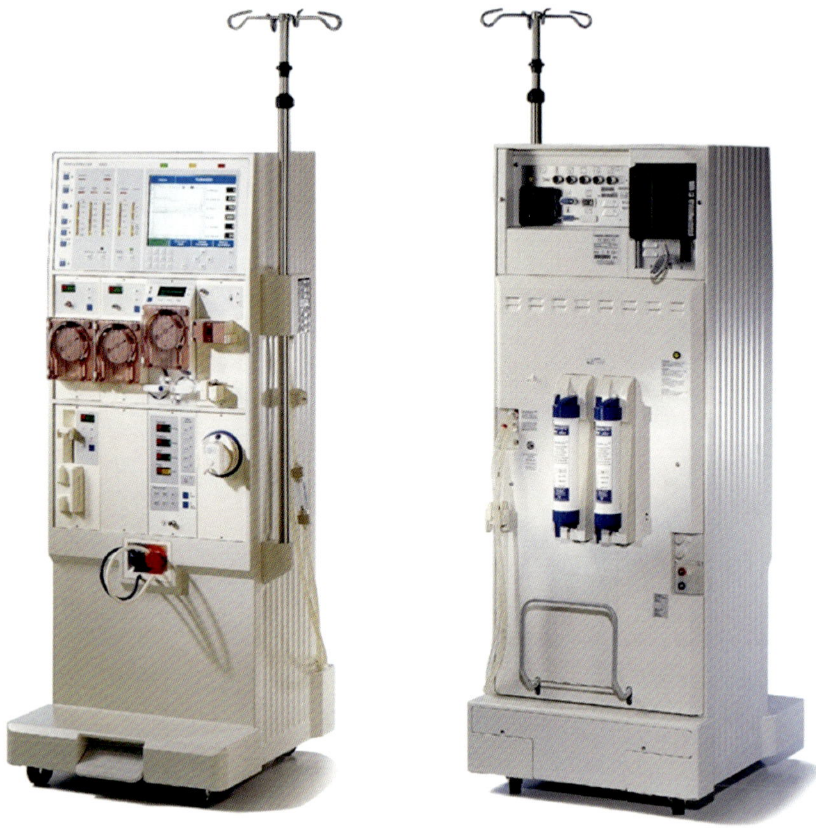

Fig. 5. Evolution of the online HDF machine with the 4008 series.

laboratory testing. By the way, on-line HDF techniques opened a new approach in the regulatory field of pharmacopoeia regarding intravenous fluids and solutions; acceptance of this approach is a matter which is not yet solved everywhere today. Water treatment systems representing a key and sensitive component for on-line methods clearly benefited from this dynamic and now deliver improved end-products. Ultrapure water is a recognized prerequisite for on-line methods but is also strongly recommended for all hemodialysis modalities by most international best practices guidelines [46]. Interestingly, water treatment and distribution systems, as a part of dialysis treatment chain, may be certified by European Community.

Several studies have shown that HDF provides significantly higher clearances than high-flux HD, both for small and middle molecule solutes [47–50]. *Phosphate* removal is increased by 15–20% over a weekly mass balance, allowing a reduction in the required amount of oral phosphate binders

[51–54]. *β_2-Microglobulin* is also more effectively removed by HDF therapies [55–57]. Due to the significantly enhanced clearance of middle molecule, HDF achieves a significant decline of circulating β_2-microglobulin concentrations over a mid-term period [58, 59]. *Leptin* (16 kDa) is a protein-bound uremic toxin that accumulates in chronic kidney disease and is implicated in malnutrition and anorexia [60]. Free leptin is effectively removed by HDF, resulting in reduced circulating concentrations in HDF-treated patients [61, 62]. *Cytokine* removal has been reported with high-flux convective therapies, both in acute and chronic ESRD patients [63]. Anti-inflammatory effects of on-line HDF have been shown in several prospective studies and are characterized by reductions in the number of pro-inflammatory monocytes and acute phase proteins [64–66]. Circulating concentrations of *oxidation-derived products (AGEs and AOPPs)* are reduced in diabetic and non-diabetic CKD patients treated by high-efficiency HDF [67]. *3-Carboxy-4-methyl-5-propyl-2-furanpropionic acid* (CMPF), a protein-bound erythropoietic inhibitor, can be reduced in HDF, particularly when using protein-leaking high-flux membranes [68, 69]. Free *p-cresyl sulfate or indoxyl sulfate*, protein-bound endothelial toxin compounds [70], are poorly removed during high-efficiency HDF [71, 72].

Clinical benefits of HDF have been underlined in treated patients in several studies. Improvement of clinical tolerance is frequently reported with convective therapies. The incidence of hypotensive episodes is reduced in HDF and HF therapies [73]. Maltolerance (nausea, vomiting, cramps, headache, etc.) of sessions is also reduced with high-efficiency HDF. Post-dialysis fatigue is less frequently observed with convective therapies. These properties are particularly advantageous for the treatment of elderly, diabetic and cardiovascular 'high-risk' patients. Better blood pressure control with reduced occurrence of cardiac events has been reported in two observational studies [74, 75]. Recent studies have shown that high-flux therapy and HDF modalities contributed to better preservation of residual renal function over time than conventional HD [76]. Anemia appears to be more easily corrected in HDF-treated patients. Although this fact remains still controversial [77], anemia correction tends to be facilitated in HDF-treated patients while the weekly EPO dose is reduced [78]. In the context of inflammatory cachexia, enhancing convective clearances is associated with an improvement of nutritional parameters (dry weight) and somatic proteins (albumin) [79, 80]. β_2-Microglobulin amyloidosis was a major concern in long-term HD therapy 20 years ago, but has virtually vanished with the regular use of new high-flux convective therapies and ultrapure dialysis fluid [81]. More interestingly, it has been recently shown that daily HDF promotes children growth, catching up to normal growth curve in this population [82]. To our knowledge, this was the first study to show that growth in CKD children could be recovered, virtually to the normal growth curve, by renal replacement therapy.

Reduced mortality of HDF-treated patients is more difficult to ascertain. Large cohort studies indicate that mortality is reduced by about 35% in HDF-treated patients even accounting for confounding factors (age, Kt/V, comorbidities, etc.), while small prospective studies did not find significant differences [83–85]. This will probably be solved in the near future by prospective, randomized, controlled studies. Two recent randomized, controlled studies (the Turkish HDF and the Contrast studies) were reported at the last ERA-EDTA congress. Both indicated significant survival benefits only for HDF-treated patients receiving large volumes of substitution fluid (17–20 liters per session) [86, 87]. This observation is of particular interest for two reasons: on the one hand, it confirms the previous findings of the DOPPS study that identified the major role of large volumes of substitution in patient survival, and on the other it raises concern regarding the true convective dialysis dose required to influence patient survival. According to findings of these studies, the concept of convective dialysis dose should be seriously considered as an add-on in the quest for dialysis adequacy.

What Does the Future Hold for On-Line Hemodiafiltration?

Despite the fact that there are still open questions, today on-line HDF offers the best option available for renal replacement therapy in chronic kidney disease patients [88]. On-line HDF is a safe and very efficient treatment modality that is associated with better patient outcomes. On-line HDF is an economically viable alternative treatment modality providing unlimited fluid replacement possibilities. Furthermore, it is a technique that is quite open for the development of new therapeutic strategies. On-line HDF has anti-inflammatory effects that are beneficial and protective for dialysis patients. Daily or nocturnal on-line HDF treatment schedules offer appealing new avenues for more physiological treatment. In addition, the access to sterile, apyrogenic, electrolytic fluid may facilitate development of automated dialysis machines for self-care or home therapy. Automated priming, rinsing of the blood circuit and volume repletion during dialysis sessions would be clearly facilitated by this option. New technical developments in HDF machines will also probably contribute to optimizing volume of substitution and favoring delivery of higher convective dialysis doses.

Conclusions

On-line HDF today offers the best renal replacement therapy option for chronic kidney disease patients, virtually at the same cost of contemporary high-flux HD. So why not offer on-line HDF to all end-stage kidney disease patients? It is a promising wager on a future of renal replacement therapy with improved patient survival and enhanced quality of patient life.

References

1 Babb AL, Ahmad S, Bergström J, Scribner BH: The middle molecule hypothesis in perspective. Am J Kidney Dis 1981;1:46–50.

2 Gotch FA, Sargent JA: A mechanistic analysis of the National Cooperative Dialysis Study (NCDS). Kidney Int 1985;28:526.

3 Daugirdas JT, Depner TA: A nomogram approach to hemodialysis urea modeling. Am J Kidney Dis 1994;23:33.

4 K/DOQI Clinical Practice Guidelines and Clinical Practice Recommendations 2006 Updates Hemodialysis adequacy Peritoneal Dialysis Adequacy Vascular Access. Am J Kidney Dis 2006;48(suppl 1):S1.

5 Vanholder R, Baurmeister U, Brunet P, Cohen G, Glorieux G, Jankowski J, European Uremic Toxin Work Group: A bench to bedside view of uremic toxins. J Am Soc Nephrol 2008;19:863–870.

6 Kessler M, Canaud B, Pedrini L, Tattersall J, Marten Ter Wee P, Vanholder R, Wanner C: Section III. Biocompatibility. EBPG Expert Group on Haemodialysis. Nephrol Dial Transplant 2002;17(suppl 7):32–44.

7 Tolchin N, Roberts JL, Hayashi J, Lewis EJ: Metabolic consequences of high mass-transfer hemodialysis. Kidney Int 1977;11:366–378.

8 Leunissen KM, Kooman JP, van Kuijk W, van der Sande F, Luik AJ, van Hooff JP: Preventing haemodynamic instability in patients at risk for intra-dialytic hypotension. Nephrol Dial Transplant 1996;11(suppl 2):11–15.

9 Selby NM, McIntyre CW: The acute cardiac effects of dialysis. Semin Dial 2007;20:220–228.

10 Kjellstrand CM, Evans RL, Petersen RJ, Shideman JR, von Hartitzsch B, Buselmeier TJ: The 'unphysiology' of dialysis: a major cause of dialysis side effects? Kidney Int Suppl 1975;2:30–34.

11 Cibulka R, Racek J: Metabolic disorders in patients with chronic kidney failure. Physiol Res 2007;56:697–705.

12 Chapman GV, Ward RA, Farrell PC: Separation and quantification of the 'middle molecules' in uremia. Kidney Int 1980;17:82–88.

13 Vanholder R, Glorieux G, De Smet R, Lameire N, European Uremic Toxin Work Group: New insights in uremic toxins. Kidney Int Suppl 2003;84:S6–S10.

14 Thomas M, Moriyama K, Ledebo I: AN69: Evolution of the World's First High Permeability Membrane. Contrib Nephrol. Basel, Karger, 2011, vol 173, pp 119–129.

15 Bowry SK, Gatti E, Vienken J: Contribution of polysulfone membranes to the success of convective dialysis therapies. Contrib Nephrol. Basel, Karger, 2011, vol 173, pp 110–118.

16 Ronco C, Bowry SK, Brendolan A, Crepaldi C, Soffiati G, Fortunato A, Bordoni V, Granziero A, Torsello G, La Greca G: Hemodialyzer: from macro-design to membrane nanostructure; the case of the FX-class of hemodialyzers. Kidney Int Suppl 2002;80:126–142.

17 Graefe U, Milutinovich J, Follette WC, Vizzo JE, Babb AL, Scribner BH: Less dialysis-induced morbidity and vascular instability with bicarbonate in dialysate. Ann Intern Med 1978;88:332–336.

18 Zelman A, White M, Acker K, Neal T, Parsons R, Gisser D: A simple method for incorporating single pass dialysate delivery and controlled ultrafiltration with the RP-6 high-flux dialyzer. J Dial 1979;3:219–235.

19 Tetta C, Roy T, Gatti E, Cerutti S: The rise of hemodialysis machines: new technologies in minimizing cardiovascular complications. Expert Rev Cardiovasc Ther 2011;9:155–164.

20 Gordon SM, Oettinger CW, Bland LA, Oliver JC, Arduino MJ, Aguero SM, McAllister SK, Favero MS, Jarvis WR: Pyrogenic reactions in patients receiving conventional, high-efficiency, or high-flux hemodialysis treatments with bicarbonate dialysate containing high concentrations of bacteria and endotoxin. J Am Soc Nephrol 1992;2:1436–1444.
21 Pegues DA, Oettinger CW, Bland LA, Oliver JC, Arduino MJ, Aguero SM, McAllister SK, Gordon SM, Favero MS, Jarvis WR: A prospective study of pyrogenic reactions in hemodialysis patients using bicarbonate dialysis fluids filtered to remove bacteria and endotoxin. J Am Soc Nephrol 1992;3:1002–1007.
22 Lonnemann G, Koch KM: Beta-2-microglobulin amyloidosis: effects of ultrapure dialysate and type of dialyzer membrane. J Am Soc Nephrol 2002;13(suppl 1):S72–S77.
23 Lonnemann G: Should ultra-pure dialysate be mandatory? Nephrol Dial Transplant 2000;15(suppl 1):55–59.
24 Canaud B, Granger-Vallée A: Should ultrapure dialysate be part of standard therapy in hemodialysis? Semin Dial 2011;24:426–427.
25 Maduell F, Navarro V, Cruz MC, Torregrosa E, Garcia D, Simon V, Ferrero JA: Osteocalcin and myoglobin removal in on-line hemodiafiltration versus low- and high-flux hemodialysis. Am J Kidney Dis 2002;40:582–589.
26 Martín-Malo A, Aljama P: On-line hemodiafiltration reduces the proinflammatory CD14+CD16+ monocyte-derived dendritic cells: a prospective, crossover study. J Am Soc Nephrol 2006;17:2315–2321.
27 Henderson LW, Beans E: Successful production of sterile pyrogen-free electrolyte solution by ultrafiltration. Kidney Int 1978;14:522–525.
28 Henderson LW, Sanfelippo ML, Beans E: 'On line' preparation of sterile pyrogen-free electrolyte solution. Trans Am Soc Artif Intern Organs 1978;24:465–467.
29 Henderson LW: Hemofiltration and the middle molecule. Blood Purif 1999;17:175–177.
30 Quellhorst E: Long-term follow-up in chronic hemofiltration. Int J Artif Organs 1983;6:115–120.
31 Baldamus CA, Quellhorst E: Outcome of long-term hemofiltration. Kidney Int Suppl 1985;17:S41–S46.
32 Ramperez P, Beau MC, Deschodt G, Flavier JL, Nilsson L, Mion C, Shaldon S: Economic preparation of sterile pyrogen-free infusate for haemofiltration. Proc Eur Dial Transplant Assoc 1981;18:293–296.
33 Shaldon S, Beau MC, Deschodt G, Flavier JL, Nilsson L, Ramperez P, Mion C: Three years of experience with on-line preparation of sterile pyrogen-free infusate for haemofiltration. Contrib Nephrol. Basel, Karger, 1982, vol 32, pp 161–164.
34 Shaldon S, Beau MC, Deschodt G, Flavier JL, Nilsson L, Ramperez P, Mion C: Three years of experience with on-line preparation of sterile pyrogen-free infusate for hemofiltration. Int J Artif Organs 1983;6:25–26.
35 Canaud B, Flavier JL, Argilés A, Stec F, N'Guyen QV, Bouloux C, Garred LJ, Mion C: Hemodiafiltration with on-line production of substitution fluid: long-term safety and quantitative assessment of efficacy. Contrib Nephrol. Basel, Karger, 1994, vol 108, pp 12–22.
36 Canaud B, Imbert E, Kaaki M, Assounga A, N'Guyen QV, Stec F, Garred LJ, Boström M, Mion C: Clinical and microbiological evaluation of a postdilutional hemofiltration system with in-line production of substitution fluid. Blood Purif 1990;8:160–170.
37 Canaud B, Araujo A, Sany C, Farrell PC, Garred LJ, Shaldon S, Mion C: A urea kinetic model for haemofiltration. Life Support Syst 1985;3:15–25.
38 Leber HW, Wizemann V, Goubeaud G, Rawer P, Schutterle G: Hemodiafiltration: a new alternative to hemofiltration and conventional hemodialysis. Artif Organs 1978;2:150–153.
39 Canaud B, N'Guyen QV, Lagarde C, Stec F, Polaschegg HD, Mion C: Clinical evaluation of a multipurpose dialysis system adequate for hemodialysis or for postdilution hemofiltration/hemodiafiltration with on-line preparation of substitution fluid from dialysate. Contrib Nephrol. Basel, Karger, 1985, vol 46, pp 184–186.

40 Canaud BJ: Changing paradigms of renal replacement therapy in chronic kidney disease patients: ultrapure dialysis fluid and high-efficiency hemodiafiltration for all? Kidney Int 2009;76:591–593.

41 Polaschegg HD, Roy T: Technical aspects of online hemodiafiltration. Contrib Nephrol. Basel, Karger, 2007, vol 158, pp 68–79.

42 Canaud B, Bosc JY, Leray-Moragues H, Stec F, Argiles A, Leblanc M, Mion C: On-line haemodiafiltration. Safety and efficacy in long-term clinical practice. Nephrol Dial Transplant 2000;15(suppl 1):60–67.

43 Canaud B, N'Guyen QV, Polito C, Stec F, Mion C: Hemodiafiltration with on-line production of bicarbonate infusate. A new standard for high-efficiency, low-cost dialysis in elderly and uncompliant patients. Contrib Nephrol. Basel, Karger, 1989, vol 74, pp 91–100.

44 Canaud B: Online hemodiafiltration. Technical options and best clinical practices. Contrib Nephrol. Basel, Karger, 2007, vol 158, pp 110–122.

45 Roy T: Technical and microbiological safety of online hemodiafiltration: a European perspective. Semin Dialysis 1999;12:S81–S87.

46 Canaud B, Mion C: Water treatment for contemporary hemodialysis; in Jacobs C, Kjellstrand CM, Koch KM, Winchester JF (eds): Replacement of Renal Function by Dialysis, ed 4. Dordrecht, Kluwer Academic, 1996, vol 8, pp 232–255.

47 Canaud B, Bosc JY, Leblanc M, Garred LJ, Vo T, Mion C: Evaluation of high-flux hemodiafiltration efficiency using an on-line urea monitor. Am J Kidney Dis 1998;31:74–80.

48 Shinzato T, Kobayakawa H, Maeda K: Comparison of various treatment modes in terms of β_2-microglobulin removal: hemodialysis, hemofiltration, and push/pull HDF. Artif Organs 1989;13:66–70.

49 Vanholder R, Meert N, Schepers E, Glorieux G: From uremic toxin retention to removal by convection: do we know enough? Contrib Nephrol. Basel, Karger, 2008, vol 161, pp 125–131.

50 Santoro A, Ferramosca E, Mancini E, Monari C, Varasani M, Sereni L, Wratten M: Reverse mid-dilution: new way to remove small and middle molecules as well as phosphate with high intrafilter convective clearance. Nephrol Dial Transplant 2007;22:2000–2005.

51 Lornoy W, De Meester J, Becaus I, Billiouw JM, Van Malderen PA, Van Pottelberge M: Impact of convective flow on phosphorus removal in maintenance hemodialysis patients. J Ren Nutr 2006;16:47–53.

52 Zehnder C, Gutzwiller JP, Renggli K: Hemodiafiltration: a new treatment option for hyperphosphatemia in hemodialysis patients. Clin Nephrol 52:152, 1999.

53 Penne EL, van der Weerd NC, van den Dorpel MA, Grooteman MP, Lévesque R, Nubé MJ, Bots ML, Blankestijn PJ, ter Wee PM, CONTRAST Investigators: Short-term effects of online hemodiafiltration on phosphate control: a result from the randomized controlled Convective Transport Study (CONTRAST). Am J Kidney Dis 2010;55:77–87.

54 Davenport A, Gardner C, Delaney M, on behalf of the Pan Thames Renal Audit Group: The effect of dialysis modality on phosphate control: haemodialysis compared to haemodiafiltration. The Pan Thames Renal Audit. Nephrol Dial Transplant 2010;25:897–901.

55 Lornoy W, Becaus I, Billiouw JM, et al: On-line haemodiafiltration. Remarkable removal of β_2-microglobulin. Long-term clinical observations. Nephrol Dial Transplant 2000;15(suppl 1):49.

56 Maduell F, del Pozo C, Garcia H, et al: Change from conventional haemodiafiltration to on-line haemodiafiltration. Nephrol Dial Transplant 1999;14:1202.

57 Padrini R, Canova C, Conz P, Mancini E, Rizzioli E, Santoro A: Convective and adsorptive removal of β_2-microglobulin during predilutional and postdilutional hemofiltration. Kidney Int 2005;68:2331–2337.

58 Locatelli F, Mastrangelo F, Redaelli B, et al: Effects of different membranes and dialysis technologies on patient treatment tolerance and nutritional parameters. The Italian Cooperative Dialysis Study Group. Kidney Int 1996;50:1293.

59 Susantitaphong P, Tiranathanagul K, Katavetin P, Townamchai N, Praditpornsilpa K, Tungsanga K, Eiam-Ong S: Efficacy of convective-controlled double high-flux hemodiafiltration versus on-line hemodiafiltration: one-year prospective study. Blood Purif 2010;29:35–43.

60 Mandolfo S, Borlandelli S, Imbasciati E: Leptin and β_2-microglobulin kinetics with three different dialysis modalities. Int J Artif Organs 2006;29:949–955.

61 Widjaja A, Kielstein JT, Horn R, et al: Free serum leptin but not bound leptin concentrations are elevated in patients with end-stage renal disease. Nephrol Dial Transplant 2000;15:846.

62 Kim S, Oh KH, Chin HJ, Na KY, Kim YS, Chae DW, Ahn C, Han JS, Kim S, Joo KW: Effective removal of leptin via hemodiafiltration with on-line endogenous reinfusion therapy. Clin Nephrol 2009;72:442–448.

63 Tetta C, Bellomo R, D'Intini V, et al: Do circulating cytokines really matter in sepsis? Kidney Int Suppl 2003;84:S69.

64 Van Tellingen A, Grooteman MP, Schoorl M, et al: Intercurrent clinical events are predictive of plasma C-reactive protein levels in hemodialysis patients. Kidney Int 2001;62:632.

65 Canaud B, Wizemann V, Pizzarelli F, et al: Cellular interleukin-1 receptor antagonist production in patients receiving on-line haemodiafiltration therapy. Nephrol Dial Transplant 2001;16:2181.

66 Carracedo J, Merino A, Nogueras S, Carretero D, Berdud I, Ramírez R, Tetta C, Rodríguez M, Martín-Malo A, Aljama P: On-line hemodiafiltration reduces the proinflammatory CD14+CD16+ monocyte-derived dendritic cells: a prospective, crossover study. J Am Soc Nephrol 2006;17:2315–2321.

67 Stein G, Franke S, Mahiout A, et al: Influence of dialysis modalities on serum AGE levels in end-stage renal disease patients. Nephrol Dial Transplant 2001;16:999.

68 Niwa T, Asada H, Tsutsui S, et al: Efficient removal of albumin-bound furancarboxylic acid by protein-leaking hemodialysis. Am J Nephrol 1995;15:463.

69 Kawano Y, Takaue Y, Kuroda Y, et al: Effect of alleviation of renal anemia by hemodialysis using the high-flux dialyzer BK-F. Kidney Dial 1994;200.

70 Meijers BK, Van Kerckhoven S, Verbeke K, Dehaen W, Vanrenterghem Y, Hoylaerts MF, Evenepoel P: The uremic retention solute *p*-cresyl sulfate and markers of endothelial damage. Am J Kidney Dis 2009;54:891–901.

71 Bammens B, Evenepoel P, Verbeke K, Vanrenterghem Y: Removal of the protein-bound solute *p*-cresol by convective transport: a randomized crossover study. Am J Kidney Dis 2004;44:278–285.

72 Krieter DH, Hackl A, Rodriguez A, Chenine L, Moragues HL, Lemke HD, Wanner C, Canaud B: Protein-bound uraemic toxin removal in haemodialysis and post-dilution haemodiafiltration. Nephrol Dial Transplant 2010;25:212–218.

73 Altieri P, Sorba G, Bolasco P, Asproni E, Ledebo I, Cossu M, Ferrara R, Ganadu M, Cadinu F, Serra G, Cabiddu G, Sau G, Casu D, Passaghe M, Bolasco F, Pistis R, Ghisu T, Second Sardinian Multicentre Study: Predilution haemofiltration – the Second Sardinian Multicentre Study: comparisons between haemofiltration and haemodialysis during identical Kt/V and session times in a long-term cross-over study. Nephrol Dial Transplant 2001;16:1207–1213.

74 Mion M, Kerr PG, Argiles A, Canaud B, Flavier JL, Mion C: Haemodiafiltration in high-cardiovascular-risk patients. Nephrol Dial Transplant 1992;7:453–454.

75 Tiranathanagul K, Praditpornsilpa K, Katavetin P, Srisawat N, Townamchai N, Susantitaphong P, Tungsanga K, Eiam-Ong S: On-line hemodiafiltration in Southeast Asia: a three-year prospective study of a single center. Ther Apher Dial 2009;13:56–62.

76 McKane W, Chandna SM, Tattersall JE, et al: Identical decline of residual renal function in high-flux biocompatible hemodialysis and CAPD. Kidney Int 2002;61:256.

77 Locatelli F, Del Vecchio L: Dialysis adequacy and response to erythropoietic agents: what is the evidence base? Nephrol Dial Transplant 2003;18(suppl 8):viii, 29–35.

78 Vaslaki L, Major L, Berta K, Karatson A, Misz M, Pethoe F, Ladanyi E, Fodor B, Stein G, Pischetsrieder M, Zima T, Wojke R, Gauly A, Passlick-Deetjen J: On-line haemodiafiltration versus haemodialysis: stable haematocrit with less erythropoietin and improvement of other relevant blood parameters. Blood Purif 2006;24:163–173.

79 Muñoz R, Gallardo I, Valladares E, Saracho R, Martínez I, Ocharan J, Montenegro J: Online hemodiafiltration: four years of clinical experience. Hemodial Int 2006;10(suppl 1):S28–S32.

80 Fischbach M, Dheu C, Seuge L, Orfanos N: Hemodialysis and nutritional status in children: malnutrition and cachexia. J Ren Nutr 2009;19:91–94.

81 Schwalbe S, Holzhauer M, Schaeffer J, Galanski M, Koch KM, Floege J: Beta-2-microglobulin-associated amyloidosis: a vanishing complication of long-term hemodialysis? Kidney Int 1997;52:1077–1083.

82 Fischbach M, Terzic J, Menouer S, Dheu C, Seuge L, Zalosczic A: Daily on-line haemodiafiltration promotes catch-up growth in children on chronic dialysis. Nephrol Dial Transplant 2010;25:867–873.

83 Canaud B, Bragg-Gresham JL, Marshall MR, Desmeules S, Gillepsie BW? Depner T, Klassen P, Port F: Patients receiving hemodiafiltration or hemofiltration have lower mortality risk than patients receiving hemodialysis without replacement fluid in Europe: The Dialysis Outcomes and Practice Patterns Study (DOPPS). J Am Soc Nephrol 2004;14:31A.

84 Jirka T, Cesare S, Di Benedetto A, Perera Chang M, Ponce P, Richards N, Tetta C, Vaslaky L: Mortality risk for patients receiving hemodiafiltration versus hemodialysis. Kidney Int 2006;70:1524.

85 Vilar E, Fry AC, Wellsted D, Tattersall JE, Greenwood RN, Farrington K: Long-term outcomes in online hemodiafiltration and high-flux hemodialysis: a comparative analysis. Clin J Am Soc Nephrol 2009;4:1944–1953.

86 Ercan O, Gulay A, Ebru S, et al: Comparison of postdilution on-line hemodiafiltration and hemodialysis. ERA-EDTA 2011, LBCT2.

87 Grooteman M, van den Dorpel R, Bots M, Penne L, van der Weerd N, Mazairac A, Den Hoedt C, Van der Tweel I, Lévesque R, Nubé M, Ter Wee P, Blankestijn P: Online hemodiafiltration versus low-flux hemodialysis: effects on all-cause mortality and cardiovascular events in a randomized controlled trial. The convective transport study (CONTRAST). ERA-EDTA 2011, LBCT1.

88 Blankestijn PJ, Ledebo I, Canaud B: Hemodiafiltration: clinical evidence and remaining questions. Kidney Int. 2010;77:581–587.

Prof. Bernard Canaud
Nephrology, Dialysis and Intensive Care Unit
Lapeyronie University Hospital, CHRU Montpellier
375, Avenue du Doyen Giraud, FR–34295 Montpellier (France)
Tel. +33 4 67 33 84 95, E-Mail b-canaud@chu-montpellier.fr

Krick G, Ronco C (eds): On-Line Hemodiafiltration: The Journey and the Vision.
Contrib Nephrol. Basel, Karger, 2011, vol 175, pp 110–116

Evolution of the Concept of Biocompatibility and the Cardioprotective Effect of On-Line Hemodiafiltration

Rafael Ramírez · Alejandro Martín-Malo · Pedro Aljama

Nephrology Department, Hospital Reina Sofia, University of Cordoba, Cordoba, Spain

Abstract

Chronic inflammation presented by chronic kidney disease patients is accompanied by an increase in the percentage of CD14+/CD16+ monocytes. The inflammatory activity produced by these cells provokes the activation and death of endothelial cells, which suggests that these cells may play an important role in the coupling of inflammation and endothelial damage in these patients. Therefore, the reduction in CD14+/CD16+ inhibitory monocytes may constitute a therapeutic goal in the treatment of chronic kidney disease patients. The use of the most effective hemodialysis techniques such as on-line hemodiafiltration appears to be a suitable tool for achieving this objective.

Patients suffering from chronic kidney disease (CKD) present a chronic inflammatory state of moderate intensity (low-grade inflammation) that appears to play an important role in the development of endothelial damage, arteriosclerosis and other cardiovascular changes, which are the principal causes of morbidity and mortality in these patients [1].

Monocytes and Disease

In the natural course of the immune response, immunocompetent cells (mainly monocytes) generate inflammation as a rapid and efficacious response to pathogens. These cells express surface molecules such as the CD14 receptor which, once they have combined with the antigen, activate the inflammatory response controlled by cytokines and other soluble factors released by activated immune cells [2]. When the antigenic stimulus ceases, the production of inflammatory cytokines also finishes, generating an anti-inflammatory response in the course of which the activated immunocompetent cells die by apoptosis [3]. This biological mechanism guarantees a controlled response that limits the perpetuation of potentially injurious cells. However, when the antigenic stimulus persists (as occurs in CKD patients with the uremic toxins and/or the immune stimulation associated with the hemodialysis therapy), the inflammatory response is perpetuated to become a chronic inflammatory response that is damaging [4].

The inflammatory profile observed in CKD patients differs from the standard inflammation and seems to be largely dependent on mononuclear cell activity [5–7]. Chronic inflammation in these patients resembles the inflammatory response described in elderly. This inflammatory response is characterized by maintaining a moderate increase in circulating proinflammatory cytokines and the presence of a subset of monocytes with a decreased expression of the CD14 receptor and the expression of the low-affinity receptor for the immunoglobulin Fc fraction, FcγRIII (CD16) [8–10].

Chronic Inflammation and CD14+/CD16+ Monocytes

In healthy subjects, peripheral blood monocytes are a heterogeneous population of cells characterized by their high level of expression of the CD14 molecule. This molecule is the receptor of the bacterial lipopolysaccharide, which is expressed in more than 90% of peripheral blood monocytes. However, under pathological situations, a different population of monocytes increase in peripheral blood, and these irregular cells are characterized to present a variable expression of the CD14 molecule and co-express the CD16 molecule. According to the levels of expression of these molecules, at least three different subsets of monocytes have been described (fig. 1): (1) monocytes with a high level of expression of CD14, which do not express CD16 (CD14++/CD16–) that are the usual monocytes found in healthy subjects; (2) CD14++/CD16+ monocytes, a population of cells found at higher levels in patients with cardiovascular pathology (stroke, infarcts, etc.) [11], and (3) inflammatory CD14+/CD16+ monocytes that are found in patients with diseases associated with chronic inflammation including CKD patients [8–10].

A large number of studies have shown an increase in the percentage of CD14+/CD16+ monocytes in CKD patients (these may make up as much as 30% of circulating monocytes in these patients) as occurs in other pathological situations. It has been suggested that the increase in CD14+/CD16+ monocytes plays a principal role in the chronic inflammatory disease associated with CKD, in contrast to that observed in the usual CD14++/

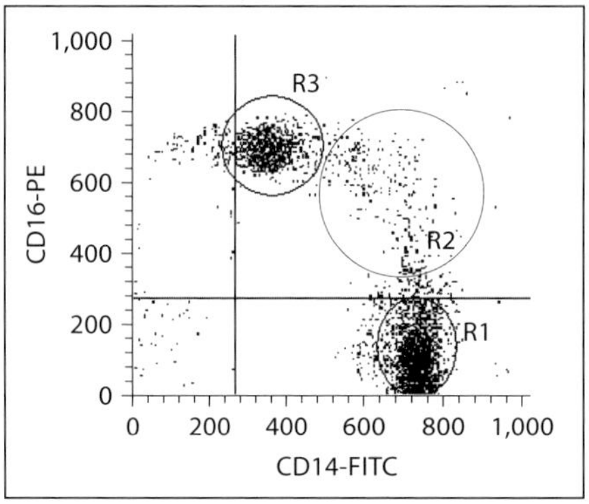

Fig. 1. Representative flow cytometry analysis of CD14 monocytes in a CKD patient. The CD14++/CD16– cells (R1) were defined as monocytes expressing CD14, but not CD16 (lower right quadrant). The CD14++/CD16– cells (R2) were defined as monocytes expressing CD16 and either high levels of CD14 (upper right quadrant). The CD14+/CD16+ cells (R3) were defined as monocytes expressing CD16 and either low levels of CD14 (upper left quadrant). For determination of CD14/CD16 cells, monocytes, were gated and labeled using 2-color fluorescence phycoerythrin (PE)-conjugated CD16 antibody, and fluorescein isothiocyanate (FITC)-conjugated CD14. R1 = CD14++/CD16–; R2 = CD14++/CD16+; R3 = CD14+/CD16+.

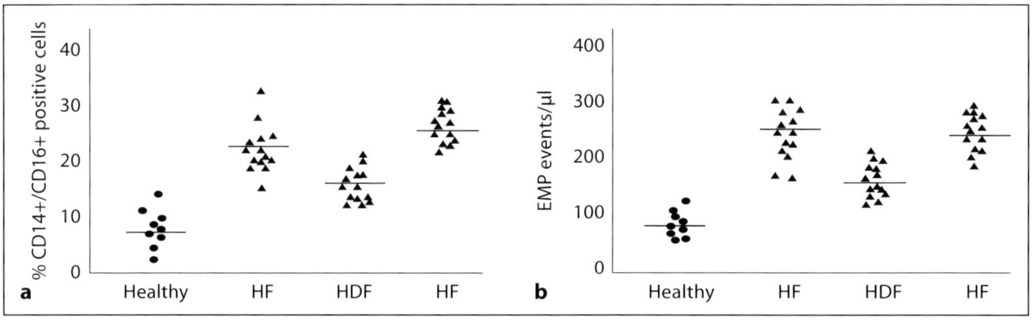

Fig. 2. Percentage of CD14+/CD16+ monocytes (**a**) and levels of endothelial microparticles (**b**) were studied by flow cytometry in 10 healthy controls and 14 CKD patients. Patients were dialyzed following the sequence: HF (basal), HDF (4 months), and HF-HD (4 months), and samples were obtained at the end of period. HF = High-flux hemodialysis; HDF = on-line hemodiafiltration.

CD16– monocytes or in CD14++/CD16+ monocytes (fig. 2). CD14+/CD16+ are activated cells that have phenotypical characteristics associated with monocyte activation, such as high expression of HLA-DR antigens or adhesion molecules, and contain high levels of preformed inflammatory cytokines in their cytoplasms [12, 13].

Why Are Inflammatory CD14+/CD16+ Cells Produced?

In addition to CKD patients, an increased number of CD14+/CD16+ cells are present in the elderly and in patients with chronic inflammation. So the question arises why such cells are produced. Recent studies performed by our group have demonstrated that CD14+/CD16+ monocytes are a population that have differentiated from CD14++/CD16– monocytes [14]. CD14+/CD16+ monocytes are generated when monocytes are repeatedly stimulated and maintained in an environment rich in proinflammatory cytokines, and these differentiated CD14+/CD16+ monocytes exhibit characteristics of senescent cells (low telomeres and expression of senescence associated enzymes such as the β-galactosidase). These data have led us to postulate that CD14+/CD16+ monocytes are activated cells that in the presence of maintained elevated levels of inflammatory cytokines (albeit moderately elevated) do not undergo apoptosis, prolong their survival and become senescent cells with a modified phenotype and functional activity.

Role Played by CD14+/CD16+ Monocytes in Endothelial Damage

Unlike what occurs with CD14++/CD16+ monocytes, whose activity is related to cardiovascular disease, inflammatory CD14+/CD16+ monocytes appear to be involved in the endothelial damage which is usually presented by elderly people and CKD or other chronic inflamed patients [15, 16]. In vitro the inflammatory response promoted by CD14+/CD16+ monocytes induced increased oxidative stress and apoptosis in endothelial cells [13]. In CKD patients, CD14+/CD16+ correlated with endothelial damage markers such as the plasma levels of endothelial microparticles or the number of reparative endothelial progenitor cells [16–18]. Additionally, the CD14+/CD16+ inflammatory monocytes exhibit high expression of adhesion molecules or chemokines such as CX3CR1, CCRS and CCR7, which facilitate the interaction between these inflammatory monocytes and the endothelium to generate a local inflammatory response that induces increased oxidative stress and apoptosis of endothelial cells [14, 19].

CD14+/CD16+ Inflammatory Monocytes in CKD Patients

As indicated above, several studies have reported that hemodialysis patients presented a higher percentage of proinflammatory CD14+/CD16+ monocytes than the healthy subjects. However there is little information about the percentage of these cells in other CKD populations such are CKD4–5 patients or CKD patients dialyzed with other techniques such as peritoneal dialysis (PD). In a recent study [19] we observed that, compared with healthy subjects, CKD4–5 patients have an increased percentage of CD14+/CD16+ monocytes (3.9 ± 1.1 in controls versus 7.7 ± 1.2% in CKD). It is important to highlight that the percentage of these cells in patients who initiate hemodialysis increased to 18.9 ± 3.5%. Interestingly, the percentage of CD14+/CD16+ cells in PD patients (3.6 ± 1.3%) was similar to that observed in healthy subjects, and no significant differences were observed when PD patients were analyzed according to their renal residual function (2.2 ± 1.5% in PD-RRF >1 and 4.3 ± 2.1% in PD-RRF ≤1).

Cardioprotective Effect of On-Line Hemodiafiltration

These data suggest that at least partially the increase in CD14+/CD16+ cells observed in CKD patients may be associated with the hemodialysis treatment. In the course of the past few years, significant advances have been made in hemodialysis therapy, particularly, after the introduction of convective therapies, such as on-line HDF, and different studies have been performed in order to analyze whether the beneficial effect of on-line HDF might be at least partially mediated by modulating the inflammatory response associated to CD14+/CD16+ monocytes. These reports showed a reduction in the percentage of CD14+/CD16+ monocytes in patients treated with on-line HDF [20–23]. Furthermore, we have reported that the reduction in CD14+/CD16+ monocytes observed in patients treated with on-line HDF is associated with a decrease in markers of endothelial damage [21], in a process that seems clearly dependent on the convective transport, and when these patients return to the high-flux techniques, the numbers of CD16 + CD14 + rise [20, 21]. Therefore, the beneficial effect of the on-line HDF seems to be related with the convective transport, and not with the biocompatibility of the dialysis membrane [16, 21].

Despite the improvement in microinflammation and endothelial damage observed in these patients, the levels of CD14+/CD16+ cells in these patients do not return to the values showed by healthy subjects. Recent studies, such as the one presented by Hung et al. [24] using anakinra, showed that these therapeutics drugs may modulate the inflammatory activity mediated by monocytes in CKD patients. Furthermore, we have preliminary data suggesting that therapeutic agents such as the angiotensin II receptor antagonists may prevent at least in vitro the differentiation of CD14+/CD16+ cells. Whether the combination of high convective transport with these drugs may eventually normalize CD14+/CD16+ cells in CKD patients constitutes a matter which remains unresolved.

Acknowledgments

This work was supported by grants from Fondo de Investigación Sanitaria, Instituto de Salud Carlos III (FIS PI10/00960, PI08/1038, RETICs Red Renal RD06/0016/0007),

Junta de Andalucía (JA0227/2009, JA0797-2010, P08-CTS-3797, P010-CTS-6337), and Fundación Nefrológica.

References

1 Foley RN, Parfrey PS, Sarnak MJ: Epidemiology of cardiovascular disease in chronic renal disease. J Am Soc Nephrol 1998;9:S16–S23.

2 Tacke F, Randolph GJ: Migratory fate and differentiation of blood monocyte subsets. Immunobiology 2006;211:609–618.

3 Maskrey BH, Megson IL, Whitfield PD, Rossi AG: Mechanisms of resolution of inflammation: a focus on cardiovascular disease. Arterioscler Thromb Vasc Biol 2011;31:1001–1006.

4 Meuwese CL, Stenvinkel P, Dekker FW, Carrero JJ: Monitoring of inflammation in patients on dialysis: forewarned is forearmed. Nat Rev Nephrol 2011;7:166–176.

5 Carracedo J, Ramirez R, Pintado O, Gomez-Villamandos JC, Martin-Malo A, Rodríguez M, Aljama P: Cell aggregation and apoptosis induced by hemodialysis membranes. J Am Soc Nephrol 1995;6:1586–1591.

6 Carracedo J, Ramírez R, Martin-Malo A, Rodríguez M, Aljama P: Nonbiocompatible hemodialysis membranes induce apoptosis in mononuclear cells: the role of G-proteins. J Am Soc Nephrol 1998;9:46–53.

7 Martín-Malo A, Carracedo J, Ramírez R, Rodriguez-Benot A, Soriano S, Rodriguez M, Aljama P: Effect of uremia and dialysis modality on mononuclear cell apoptosis. J Am Soc Nephrol 2000;11:936–942.

8 Nockher WA, Scherberich JE: Expanded CD14+/CD16+ monocyte subpopulation in patients with acute and chronic infections undergoing hemodialysis. Infect Immun 1998;66:2787–2790.

9 Scherberich JE, Nockher WA: Blood monocyte phenotypes and soluble endotoxin receptor CD14 in systemic inflammatory diseases and patients with chronic renal failure. Nephrol Dial Transplant 2000;15:574–578.

10 Carracedo J, Ramírez R, Martin-Malo A, Rodríguez M, Aljama P: The effect of LPS, uraemia, and haemodialysis membrane exposure on CD14 expression in mononuclear cells and its relation to apoptosis. Nephrol Dial Transplant 2002;17:428–434.

11 Rogacev KS, Seiler S, Zawada AM, Reichart B, Herath E, Roth D, Ulrich C, Fliser D, Heine GH: CD14++CD16+ monocytes and cardiovascular outcome in patients with chronic kidney disease. Eur Heart J 2011;32:84–92.

12 Ramirez R, Carracedo J, Berdud I, Carretero D, Merino A, Rodríguez M, Tetta C, Martín-Malo A, Aljama P: Microinflammation in hemodialysis is related to a preactivated subset of monocytes. Hemodial Int 2006;10(suppl 1):S24–S27.

13 Ziegler-Heitbrock L: The CD14+ CD16+ blood monocytes: their role in infection and inflammation. J Leukoc Biol 2007;81:584–592.

14 Merino A, Buendia P, Martin-Malo A, Aljama P, Ramirez R, Carracedo J: Senescent CD14+CD16+ monocytes exhibit proinflammatory and proatherosclerotic activity. J Immunol 2011;186:1809–1815.

15 Li G, Kim YJ, Mantel C, Broxmeyer HE: P-selectin enhances generation of CD14+CD16+ dendritic-like cells and inhibits macrophage maturation from human peripheral blood monocytes. J Immunol 2003;171:669–677.

16 Ramirez R, Carracedo J, Merino A, Nogueras S, Alvarez-Lara MA, Rodríguez M, Martin-Malo A, Tetta C, Aljama P: Microinflammation induces endothelial damage in hemodialysis patients: the role of convective transport. Kidney Int 2007;72:108–113.

17 Merino A, Nogueras S, García-Maceira T, Rodríguez M, Martin-Malo A, Ramirez R, Carracedo J, Aljama P: Bacterial DNA and endothelial damage in haemodialysis patients. Nephrol Dial Transplant 2008;23:3635–3642.
18 Merino A, Nogueras S, Buendía P, Ojeda R, Carracedo J, Ramirez-Chamond R, Martin-Malo A, Aljama P: Microinflammation and endothelial damage in hemodialysis. Contrib Nephrol. Basel, Karger, 2008, vol 161, pp 83–88.
19 Merino A, Portolés J, Selgas R, Ojeda R, Buendia P, Ocaña J, Bajo MA, del Peso G, Carracedo J, Ramírez R, Martín-Malo A, Aljama P: Effect of different dialysis modalities on microinflammatory status and endothelial damage. Clin J Am Soc Nephrol 2010;5:227–234.
20 Ramírez R, Carracedo J, Merino A, Soriano S, Ojeda R, Alvarez-Lara MA, Martín-Malo A, Aljama P: CD14+CD16+ monocytes from chronic kidney disease patients exhibit increased adhesion ability to endothelial cells. Contrib Nephrol. Basel, Karger, 2011, vol 171, pp 57–61.
21 Carracedo J, Merino A, Nogueras S, Carretero D, Berdud I, Ramírez R, Tetta C, Rodríguez M, Martín-Malo A, Aljama P: On-line hemodiafiltration reduces the proinflammatory CD14+CD16+ monocyte-derived dendritic cells: a prospective, crossover study. J Am Soc Nephrol 2006;17:2315–2321.
22 Rogacev KS, Seiler S, Zawada AM, Reichart B, Herath E, Roth D, Ulrich C, Fliser D, Heine GH: CD14++CD16+ monocytes and cardiovascular outcome in patients with chronic kidney disease. Eur Heart J 2011;32:84–92.
23 Kim HW, Yang HN, Kim MG, Choi HM, Jo SK, Cho WY, Kim HK: Microinflammation in hemodialysis patients is associated with increased CD14CD16+ pro-inflammatory monocytes: possible modification by on-line hemodiafiltration. Blood Purif 2011;31:281–288.
24 Hung AM, Ellis CD, Shintani A, Booker C, Ikizler TA: IL-1β receptor antagonist reduces inflammation in hemodialysis patients. J Am Soc Nephrol 2011;22:437–442.

Pedro Aljama
Nephrology Department, Hospital Universitario Reina Sofía
Avda Menendez Pidal S/N, Córdoba 14004 (Spain)
Tel. +34 011 34 957 010143
E-Mail pedro.aljama.sspa@juntadeandalucia.es

Krick G, Ronco C (eds): On-Line Hemodiafiltration: The Journey and the Vision.
Contrib Nephrol. Basel, Karger, 2011, vol 175, pp 117–128

On-Line Hemodiafiltration in the Large RISCAVID Study

Vincenzo Panichi[a] · Ciro Tetta[b]

[a]Nephrology and Dialysis Versilia Hospital, Versilia, Italy; [b]Fresenius Medical Care, Bad Homburg, Germany

Abstract

Despite significant advances in hemodialysis (HD) and medical therapy, mortality rates in patients with chronic kidney disease stage 5 (CKD-5D) remain unacceptably high, with cardiovascular (CV) mortality risk in dialysis patients being several times higher than that of a general population. The CV mortality risk of a 25- to 34-year-old dialysis patient is approximately the same as the one of an otherwise healthy person aged over 85 in the general population. HD patients are not only exposed to the various traditional risk factors valid for the general population but in addition also to the non-traditional risk factors resulting either from uremia per se or from the dialysis treatment. Our understanding of chronic inflammation in CKD-5D and of its influence in the accelerated atherosclerotic process has greatly evolved. Dialysis therapy, performed efficiently, has the potential to provide CKD-5D patients with benefits beyond the life-saving function of removal accumulated waste products and excess fluid. There is sufficient evidence to indicate that on-line hemodiafiltration has the potential to improve chronic inflammation, fluid overload, left ventricular hypertrophy, anemia and quality of life of CKD-5D patients. In the search for more effective, safer and less expensive approaches to the management of the above conditions, an innovative concept of biocompatibility should be broadened to the HD system/patient evaluation. Here, we intend to present new insights obtained from a prospective observational study (RISCAVID, 'RISchio CArdiovascolare nei pazienti afferenti all'Area Vasta In Dialisi') performed on a large HD population in the northwestern region of Tuscany, Italy, on the assessment of the different parameters of chronic inflammation and gross/CV mortality and anemia management.

The concept that inflammation underlies many diseases, once considered to be linked to degenerative processes, has revolutionized the approach to the research into the pathogenesis and new therapeutics alike. In the field of cardiovascular disease (CVD), the process of endothelial dysfunction, vascular damage and atherosclerosis is now seen as a continuum [1]. CVD is among the leading causes of morbidity and mortality in chronic kidney disease stage 5 (CKD-5D) patients on maintenance hemodialysis (HD) [2, 3]. Even patients with reducing renal function already present with signs of chronic inflammation. Once patients are on HD, the risk of cardiovascular (CV) death is approximately 30 times higher than in the general population, and still remains 10–20 times higher after stratification for age, gender, and presence of diabetes. It is now well established that inflammation plays a primary role in arterial damage in HD patients [4, 5]. Although the precise mechanisms that are responsible for inflammation in ESRD are still unclear, the uremic status per se, low-grade infection, repeated exposure to foreign surfaces and auto-oxidation products are considered as likely inciting factors in these patients [6]. Recent studies have shown that epigenetic modifications orchestrate the epithelial-mesenchymal transition and eventually fibrosis of the renal tissue. Oxidative stress, inflammation, hyperhomocysteinemia, and uremic toxins could induce epimutations in CKD. Epigenetic alterations are associated with inflammation and CVD in patients with CKD [7]. Furthermore, a variety of traditional and non-traditional risk factors such as sympathetic hyperactivity, dyslipidemia, hyperphosphatemia/hyperparathyroidism, diabetes, and smoking may activate and/or amplify the inflammatory process in CKD-5D.

Inflammatory mechanisms play a relevant role in the development and progression of atherosclerosis [8] and heart failure [9]. Epidemiological studies in the general population have shown that even minor elevations of C-reactive protein (CRP), an acute-phase reactant that markedly increases during an inflammatory response [10], predict the development of coronary heart disease and cardiac failure [11–13]. CRP may directly promote the development of atherosclerosis, through complement activation, tissue damage and activation of endothelial cells. Studies performed in CKD-5D patients showed that CRP is a strong predictor of CV death [14, 15]. The link between CRP and CV risk was initially thought to be indirect, reflecting circulating CRP only to the extent of the acute phase reaction in response to non-specific stimuli such as confounding risk factors, atherosclerosis, vascular injury, ischemia and necrosis. However, several arguments now indicate that CRP is not merely an epiphenomenon, but it is also involved in the pathogenesis of the disease.

Stenvinkel et al. [16] first convincingly showed that the malnutrition-inflammation-atherosclerosis (MIA) syndrome is associated with the highest mortality rates in CKD-5D. Their results have been confirmed and extended [17]. As reviewed by Stenvinkel and Bárány [18], there is consensus on a link between CKD-5D and inflammation. A number of studies have highlighted the association between increased inflammatory indexes and a reduced response to erythropoiesis-stimulating agents (ESAs), in particular, high CRP levels were found in HD patients requiring higher ESA doses [19, 20]. However, the association between ESA resistance and increased CRP levels [21] is still unclear. Plasma interleukin (IL)-6 rather than CRP seems to better predict outcomes in CKD-5D patients [22]. Various possible explanations may underline the advantage of IL-6 over CRP as a predictor of ESA resistance. One possibility is that IL-6, being located upstream in the cascade of events which lead to the synthesis of many acute-phase reactants, is a better marker for the inflammatory burden affecting the development of CVD [23]. A frequently-asked question is what is the contribution of HD bioincompatibility to the chronic inflammatory state? In this context, the evolution of HD technology has moved the focus from membrane bioincompatibility only to a more complex and integrated view of the HD system. The possibility that HD may be shift to a 'cardioprotective" therapy is inherent to new technologies in machines, water treatment, dialysis fluids and blood tubings.

Originally introduced as an elegant concept in 1986 [24], the 'interleukin hypothesis' was first coined to indicate the production of IL-1, the endogenous pyrogen as produced by the result of complement-activated mononuclear cells. Indeed, the interleukin hypothesis explained much more than was initially predictable. Ever since, several studies have reported an increased cytokine production secondary to blood interaction with contaminated dialysate. IL-1, tumor necrosis factor-α and mainly IL-6 are the three pro-inflammatory cytokines that are involved in the pathogenesis of HD-dependent chronic inflammation [as reviewed in 25, 26].

The proposed mechanisms include blood interaction with endotoxins from the contaminated dialysate through HD membranes. A large number of studies have greatly contributed to increasing our knowledge in the mechanisms of endotoxin transfer across the membranes. In fact, when using high permeability membranes, backfiltration and backdiffusion occur [27]. Thus, the transmembrane passage of endotoxins or other cytokine-stimulating substances occurs during HD [28]. The reduction of backfiltration of standard dialysate may reduce the plasma concentration of IL-1ra, a sensitive indicator of inflammation in HD patients [Dinarello, pers. commun., 2004], and IL-1 [17]. Studies on large groups of patients have shown that high-volume exchange hemodiafiltration (HDF), a modality in which dialysate backfiltration is minimal, is associated with significantly lower CRP plasma values [17]. Comparing in a double crossover study patients treated with high-flux and on-line HDF using ultrapure dialysate and infusate, it was shown that a significant reduction of pro-inflammatory CD14+/CD16+ mononuclear subset occurs in on-line HDF [29]. These studies emphasize that the convective component has an additional anti-inflammatory effect [30].

The new technology of pyrogen-adsorbing, non-complement activating, high-permeability synthetic membranes and dedicated machines [31], as well as the awareness of the deleterious effects derived from contamination of dialysis fluids, has reduced the clinical impact to a periodic microinflammatory stimulus. Undoubtedly, the availability of monitors for on-line HDF and its increased popularity have spurred more restrictive measures on safety issues and monitoring. Water quality is a mandatory issue. Nowadays, the consolidated, clinical experience with on-line HDF warrants well-defined procedures and leaves no space for 'experiments' in what is now routine [32, 33]. The 'hemocompatibility network' should eventually prevent the periodic microinflammation induction through the implementation of rigid protocols of disinfection and maintenance of water treatment systems and HD monitors [3].

Experience of the RISCAVID

In June 2004, a prospective observational study (RISCAVID, *'RISchio CArdiovascolare nei pazienti afferenti all'Area Vasta In Dialisi'*) was started with the aim to investigate the link between traditional and non-traditional risk factors on mortality and morbidity in a large and homogenous HD population in the northwestern region of Tuscany. 757 patients representing the whole HD population of 1,235,062 inhabitants were included. Each of the 15 dialysis facilities of this region provided at the start of the study blood samples from all patients for the determination of inflammatory markers and at the start and every 6 months data on patients' demographic characteristics, renal history, laboratory values, comorbid disease, dialysis techniques, vascular access prescriptions and outcomes (table 1).

Three papers have been published to date on the basis of the results of the RISCAVID database. The first described the role of chronic inflammation and the impact of different HD modalities on morbidity and mortality rates [34]. The second focused on the erythropoietic response to ESA treatment and the factors involved in resistance to ESA [23]. The third examined the clinical relevance of serum mineral derangements, and the impact of different therapeutic strategies on mineral metabolism and mortality [35].

Chronic Inflammation and the Impact of Different HD Modalities on Morbidity and Mortality

High levels of CRP and inflammatory cytokines and low serum albumin are strong outcome predictors in CKD-5D patients, supporting the hypothesis that chronic inflammation is an important risk factor for CV and overall mortality in this population. CRP, IL-6, IL-8 and albumin have synergic effects on CV and overall mortality. In practical terms, determination of CRP at least at the initiation of HD might be recommended to evaluate an increased

Table 1. Population, clinical and laboratory characteristics as well as HD modalities

Demographics and clinical characteristics (757 patients)	
Age, years	66 (14)
Male/female	458/296
Dialytic age, months	70 (76)
Body mass index	23.9 (4.4)
Comorbidites	
CVD	197 (26%)
Diabetes	143 (19%)
Hypertension	265 (35%)
Malignancy	106 (14%)
Systolic BP, mm Hg	135 (21)
Diastolic BP, mm Hg	74 (10)
HD modalities and parameters	
HD modalities, n (%)	
BHD/Kt/V	424 (56%)/1.39
HDF/Kt/V	205 (27%)/1.41
On-line HDF/kT/V	128 (17%)/1.43
Type of membrane, n (%)	
Modified cellulose	98 (13%)
Synthetic	659 (87%)
Laboratory parameters	
Hemoglobin, g/dl	11.6 (1.5)
Iron, μg/dl	70.4 (36)
Transferrin, mg/dl	179.9 (48.7)
Ferritin, ng/dl	496.4 (523)
TSAT, %	29.4 (17)
ERI, IU weekly/kg/g hemoglobin	11.9 (9.3)
Patients receiving ESAs, n (%)	651 (86%)
Calcium, mg/dl	9.1 (3.2)
Phosphate, mg/dl	4.8 (1.5)
iPTH, pg/dl	277 (282)
Ca × P, mg^2/dl^2	44.4 (14.8)
Total serum cholesterol, mg/dl	169.3 (47)
LDL cholesterol, mg/dl	88.9 (38.6)
Albumin, g/dl	3.7 (0.4)
CRP, mg/dl	10 (14.5)

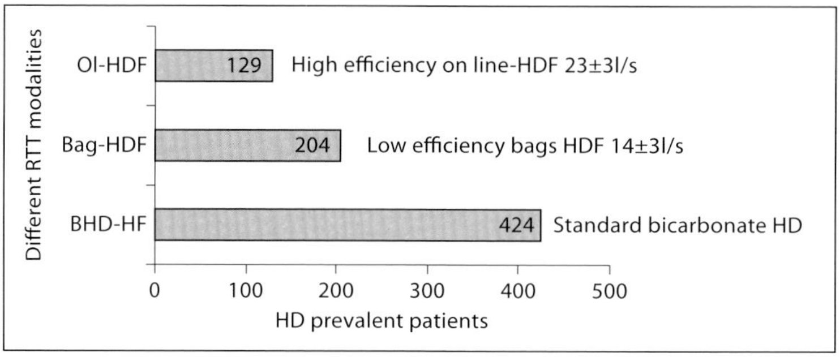

Fig. 1. RISCAVID study population according to dialysis technique.

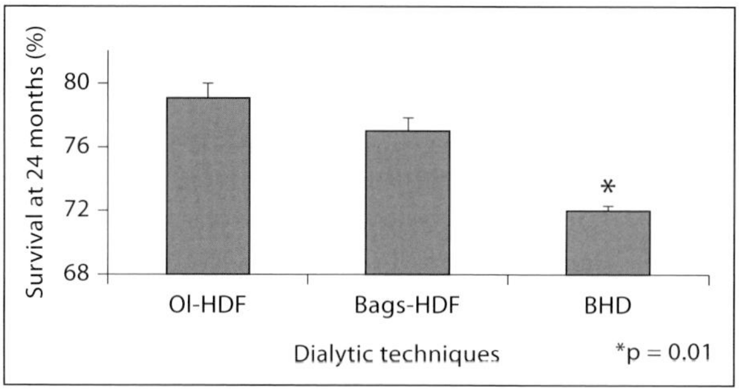

Fig. 2. Cumulative survival of patients receiving bicarbonate dialysis in comparison to patients receiving bags of HDF and on-line HDF.

risk and to appropriately adjust patient medication and care. Our study also provided information on the effect of different HD modalities on chronic inflammation and consequently on the cumulative survival. IL-6, a strong predictor for CV mortality, was found to be decreased in on-line HDF. The enhanced cumulative survival of patients receiving HDF in comparison to standard bicarbonate dialysis observed in RISCAVID (fig. 1, 2) extended the results by Canaud et al. [36] who compared the mortality of patients receiving HDF to that of patients receiving HD in a large cohort prospectively followed for 3 years in the Dialysis Outcomes and Practice Patterns Study (DOPPS) [37]. These authors showed that the mortality risk of patients receiving high-efficiency HDF was significantly lower (35%) when adjusting for differences in the comorbidity profile. However, in the DOPPS only surrogate markers of inflammation were measured, i.e. albumin and ferritin, since the measurements of CRP and cytokines had originally not been taken into account in the data collection. With respect to the DOPPS, the RISCAVID population differed from other existing studies in the high incidence of mixed convective-diffusive techniques (HDF 44% of the entire population). Of interest in our study, the difference in cumulative survival started after 15 months of observation after adjustment for age, dialysis vintage and comorbidities. At variance with the paper with Canaud et al. [36], we were not able to establish a relationship between mortality and volume exchange. Despite this limitation, HDF using sterile bags is customarily prescribed using 10–15 liters/session of reinfusion fluid while on-line HDF is performed with at least 22–25 liters/session.

EPO Resistance

Using the RISCAVID database, we investigated how anemia, ESA resistance and the plasma levels of biological markers of chronic inflammation could influence all-cause mortality and fatal/non-fatal CV events. Anemia is a common complication and predictor of mortality in CKD-5D patients [38]. A vast majority of these patients receives ESAs and resistance to this therapy is common [39]. In CKD-5D patients, anemia is linked to inflammation and oxidative stress is associated with the uremic syndrome [18]. Moreover, CKD-5D patients may require much higher than usual doses of ESAs in order to maintain the recommended hemoglobin target of ≥11 g/dl [40]. In many instances, these patients will have either an obvious or a clinically unapparent inflammatory process to account for the hyporesponsiveness to ESA replacement therapy. In this setting, the term ESA resistance has been introduced to define patients who fail to reach the target despite a higher than usual dose of ESAs or who continuously need higher doses in order to maintain it. Firstly, hemoglobin levels <11 g/dl were associated with the highest risk for all-cause mortality and fatal/non-fatal CV events while patients with hemoglobin levels >11 g/dl had the lowest all-cause mortality risk which was comparable to the reference group (no ESAs). After adjusting for confounders, hemoglobin did not affect fatal/non-fatal CV events. Other factors such as age, history of CVD, and serum albumin influenced both all-cause mortality and fatal/non-fatal CV events; CRP was a predictor of all-cause mortality but not of fatal/non-fatal CV events; conversely total cholesterol predicted fatal/non-fatal CV events but not all-cause mortality. Of note, Kt/V, pre-HD blood urea, HD vs. HDF, smoking and pulse pressure increased the relative risk of all-cause mortality and/or of fatal/non-fatal CV events at the univariate but not at the multivariate analysis. Moreover, CRP and IL-6 did not increase the relative risk of fatal/non-fatal CV events. Furthermore, the degree of ESA resistance showed a highly significant correlation with all-cause and CV mortality. In our model, the predictive power of the degree of resistance was higher than that of hemoglobin. Moreover, hyporesponders were the oldest and had the lowest serum albumin and TSAT levels as well as the highest plasma IL-6 values. However, serum albumin is not a valid marker of protein energy wasting given its dependence on inflammation, urinary albumin losses and hydration status. Finally, factors that influenced the degree of ESA resistance were low serum albumin, IL-6, as well as TSAT and therapy with sevelamer, statins and ESA. Of note, CRP did not influence the ESA Resistance Index (ERI).

Although the study was confirmatory, the results are based on a rather large cohort of a rather homogenous HD population. The prognostic significance of resistance to ESAs has been studied before by Kilpatrick et al. [41], who showed that a greater responsiveness to ESAs is associated with improved survival. As shown by the secondary analysis of the CHOIR trial [42], patients achieving their hemoglobin target had better outcomes than those who did not. Therefore, the evaluation of the mechanisms interfering with the action of ESAs seems relevant for the determination of an appropriate anemia management.

Impact of Mineral Metabolism Derangements

In a third paper, the impact of phosphate, calcium, intact parathyroid hormone (iPTH), K/DOQI recommendations, and different therapeutic strategies for chronic kidney disease-mineral bone disorders (CKD-MBD) on CV and all-cause mortality in the RISCAVID population was reported. At study entry, according to K/DOQI guidelines, only 71 (9%) and 239 (32%) patients exhibited all four or at least three bone mineral parameters (namely Ca, Pi, Ca × Pi and iPTH) within the suggested ranges. Despite a similar prevalence, the severity of CKD-MBD appeared different to what was reported in the USA. Of interest, none of the serum biomarkers or the number of serum biomarkers within K/DOQI targets were independently associated with all-cause and CV mortality. When Pi, calcium phosphate and all-cause and CV mortality were plotted together, a U-shaped relationship was noted for both parameters (fig. 3, 4). However, adjustments for factors calcium phosphate product with Pi and calcium phosphate significantly attenuated these associations that lost statistical significance. Similar to that found by others, the CKD-MBD syndrome affects the majority calcium phosphate product of patients enrolled in the RISCAVID study. Nonetheless, though our findings are in line with what was reported in the Italian cohort of the DOPPS study, a few differences deserve consideration. When compared to the overall DOPPS study cohort, hyperphosphatemia and the use of phosphate binders is substantially less prevalent in the RISCAVID study [43, 44]. However, the lower prevalence of hyperphosphatemia might be partly accounted for by differences in race, diet, dialysis and CKD-MBD management that exist between countries. Indeed, some authors suggested women and Blacks tend to have higher levels of serum phosphate, iPTH and FGF-23. Furthermore, the greater use of convective/diffusive techniques in our study, the low-protein diet and different nutrition policies might also contribute to the low prevalence of hyperphosphatemia in Italy.

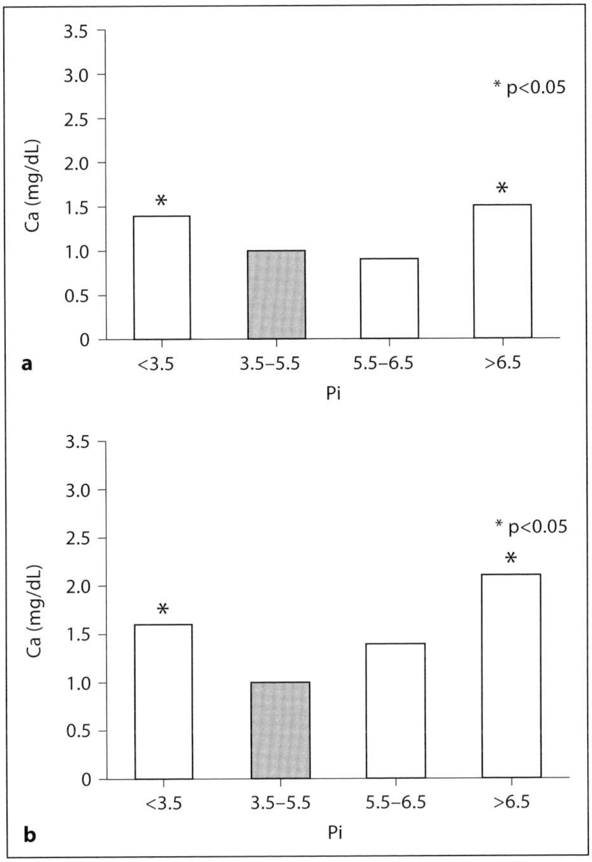

Fig. 3. Overall (**a**) and CV (**b**) mortality relative risk according to phosphate levels.

Conclusions

The RISCAVID database with both an incident and prevalent population homogenous for origin and similar practice patterns has proved to be a relevant tool for following up a large cohort over 36 months and for drawing and conclusions on the incidence and evolution of chronically inflamed patients regarding morbidity and mortality. The impact of chronic inflammation on ESA resistance has also been shown. Despite the limitations inherent to any observational study, we are continuing to accrue data on this geographical region to further extend our observations period.

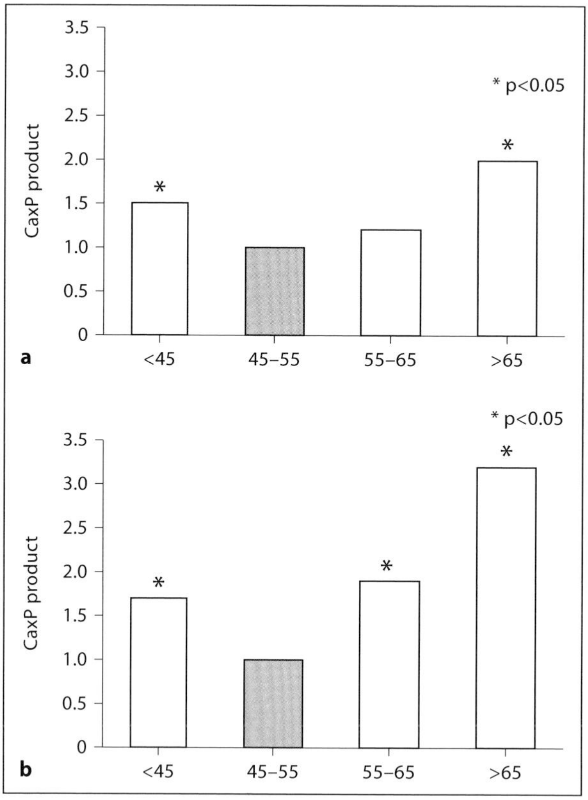

Fig. 4. Overall (**a**) and CV (**b**) mortality relative risk according to Ca x P product.

References

1 Libby P, Ridker PM, Maseri A: Inflammation and atherosclerosis. Circulation 2002;3:187–197.

2 US Renal Data System: Excerpts from the USRDS 1997 annual data report. Am J Kidney Dis 1997;30:S1–S195.

3 Parfey PS, Foley RN: The clinical epidemiology of cardiac disease in chronic renal failure. J Am Soc Nephrol 1999;10:1606–1615.

4 Stenvinkel P, Heinburger O, Paultre F, et al: Strong associations between malnutrition, inflammation and atherosclerosis in chronic renal failure. Kidney Int 1999;55:1899–1911.

5 Tripepi G, Mallamaci F, Zoccali C: Inflammation markers, adhesion molecules, and all-cause and cardiovascular mortality in patients with ESRD: searching for the best risk marker by multivariate modeling. J Am Soc Nephrol 2005(suppl 1):S83–S88.

6 Schouten WEM, Grooteman MPC, van Houte AJ, et al: Effects of dialysers and dialysate on the acute phase reaction in clinical bicarbonate dialysis. Nephrol Dial Transplant 2000;15:379–384.

7 Dwivedi RS, Herman JG, McCaffrey TA, Raj DS: Beyond genetics: epigenetic code in chronic kidney disease. Kidney Int 2011;79:23–32.

8 Ross R. Atherosclerosis: an inflammatory disease. N Engl J Med 1999;340:115–126.

9 Vasan RS, Sullivan LM, Roubenoff R, Dinarello CA, Harris T, Benjamin EJ, Sawyer DB, Wilson PW, D'Agostino RB: Inflammatory markers and risk of heart failure in elderly subjects without prior myocardial infarction: The Framingham Heart Study. Circulation 2003;107:1486–1491.
10 Ridker PM, Cushman M, Stampfer MJ, Tracy RP, Hennekens CH: Inflammation, aspirin and the risk of cardiovascular disease in apparently healthy men. N Engl J Med 1997;336:973–979.
11 Liuzzo G, Biasucci LM, Gallimore JR, Grillo RL, Rebuzzi AG, Pepys MB, Maseri A: The prognostic value of C-reactive protein and serum amyloid a protein in severe unstable angina. N Engl J Med 1994;331:417–424.
12 Lagrand WK, Visser CA, Hermens WT, Niesssen HW, Verheught FW, Wolbink J, Hack CE: C-reactive protein as a cardiovascular risk: more than an epiphenomenon? Circulation 1999;100:96–102.
13 Bhatt DL, Topol EJ: Need to test the arterial Inflammation hypothesis. Circulation 2002;106:136–140.
14 Stenvinkel P: Malnutrition and chronic inflammation as risk factors for cardiovascular disease in chronic renal failure. Blood Purif 2001;19:143–151.
15 Kaysen GA: Inflammation: cause of vascular disease and malnutrition in dialysis patients. Semin Nephrol 2004;24:431–436.
16 Stenvinkel P, Heinburger O, Paultre F, Diczfalusy U, Wang T, Berglund L, Jogestrand T: Strong associations between malnutrition, inflammation and atherosclerosis in chronic renal failure. Kidney Int 1999;55:1899–1911.
17 Panichi V, Tetta C, Rindi P, Palla R, Lonnemann G: Plasma C-reactive protein is linked to backfiltration associated interleukin-6 production. ASAIO J 1998;744:M415–M417.
18 Stenvinkel P, Bárány P: Anaemia, rHuEPO resistance, and cardiovascular disease in end-stage renal failure; links to inflammation and oxidative stress. Nephrol Dial Transplant 2002;17(suppl 5):32–37.
19 Singh AK, Coyne DW, Shapiro W, Rizkala AR: Predictors of the response to treatment in anemic haemodialysis patients with high serum ferritin and low transferring saturation. Kidney Int 2007;71:1163–1171.
20 Bradbury BD, Critchlow CV, Weir MR Stewart R, Krishnan M, Hakim RH: Impact of elevated C-reactive protein levels on erythropoiesis-stimulating agent dose and responsiveness in haemodialysis patients. Nephrol Dial Transplant 2009;24:919–925.
21 Bárány P, Divino Filho JC, Bergström J: High C-reactive protein is a strong predictor of resistance to erythropoietin in hemodialysis patients. Am J Kidney Dis 1997;29:565–568.
22 Panichi V, Maggiore U, Taccola D, Migliori M, Rizza GM, Consani C, Bertini A, Sposini-Garcia R, Rindi P, Palla R, Tetta C: Interleukin-6 is a stronger predictor of total and cardiovascular mortality than C-reactive protein in hemodialysis patients. Nephrol Dial Transplant 2004;19:1154–1160.
23 Panichi V, Rosati A, Bigazzi R, Paoletti S, Mantuano E, Beati S, Marchetti V, Bernabini G, Grazi G, Rizza GM, Migliori M, Giusti R, Lippi A, Casani A, Barsotti G, Tetta C, on behalf of the RISCAVID Study Group: Anaemia and resistance to erythropoiesis-stimulating agents as prognostic factors in haemodialysis patients: results from the RISCAVID study. Nephrol Dial Transplant 2011;26:2641–2618.
24 Bingel M, Lonnemann G, Shaldon S, Koch KM, Dinarello CA: Human interleukin-1 production during hemodialysis. Nephron 1986;43:161–163.
25 Lonnemann G: When good water goes bad: how it happens, clinical consequences and possible solutions. Blood Purif 2004;22:124–129.
26 Panichi V, Migliori M, De Pietro S, Taccola D, Andreini B, Metelli MR, Giovannini L, Palla R: The link of biocompatibility to cytokine production. Kidney Int 2000;59(suppl 76):96–103.
27 Ronco C: Fluid mechanics and cross-filtration in hollow-fiber hemodialyzers. Contrib Nephrol. Basel, Karger, 2007, vol 158, pp 34–49.
28 Tetta C, Maffei S, Cisterna B, et al: The evolution of biocompatibility: from microinflammation to microvesicles. Hemodialysis. InTech Publishers, 2011, in press.

29 Carracedo J, Merino A, Nogueras S, Carretero D, Berdud I, Ramírez R, Tetta C, Rodríguez M, Martín-Malo A, Aljama P: Online hemodiafiltration reduces the proinflammatory CD14+CD16+ monocyte-derived dendritic cells: a prospective, crossover study. J Am Soc Nephrol 2006;17:2315–2321.
30 Ramirez R, Carracedo J, Merino A, Nogueras S, Alvarez-Lara MA, Rodríguez M, Martin-Malo A, Tetta C, Aljama P: Microinflammation induces endothelial damage in hemodialysis patients: the role of convective transport. Kidney Int 2007;72:108–113.
31 Tetta C, Roy T, Gatti E, Cerutti S: The rise of hemodialysis machines: new technologies in minimizing cardiovascular complications. Expert Rev Cardiovasc Ther 2011;9:155–164.
32 Canaud B, Chenine L, Renaud S, Leray H: Optimal therapeutic conditions for online hemodiafiltration. Contrib Nephrol. Basel, Karger, 2011, vol 168, pp 28–38.
33 Cappelli G, Riccardi M, Perrone S, Bondi M, Ligabue G, Albertazzi A: Water treatment and monitor disinfection. Hemodialysis Int 2006;10(suppl 1):S13–S18.
34 Panichi V, Rizza GM, Paoletti S, Bigazzi R, Aloisi M, Barsotti G, Rindi P, Donati G, Antonelli A, Panicucci E, Tripepi G, Tetta C, Palla R, RISCAVID Study Group: Chronic inflammation and mortality in haemodialysis: effect of different renal replacement therapies. Results from the RISCAVID study. Nephrol Dial Transplant 2008;23:2337–2343.
35 Panichi V, Bigazzi R, Paoletti S, Mantuano E, Beati S, Marchetti V, Bernabini G, Grazi G, Giust R, Rosati A, Migliori M, Pasquariello A, Panicucci E, Barsotti G, Bellasi A, RISCAVID Study Group: Impact of calcium, phosphate, PTH abnormalities and management on mortality in hemodialysis: results from the RISCAVID study. J Nephrol 2010;23:556–562.
36 Canaud B, Bragg-Gresham JL, Marshall MR, Desmeules S, Gillespie BW, Depner T, Klassen P, Port FK: Mortality risk for patients receiving hemodiafiltration versus hemodialysis: European results from the DOPPS. Kidney Int 2006;69:2087–2093.
37 Goodkin DA, Young EW, Kurokawa K, Prutz KG, Levin NW: Mortality among hemodialysis patients in Europe, Japan, and the United States: case-mix effects. Am J Kidney Dis 2004;44(suppl 2):16–21.
38 Regidor DL, Kopple JD, Kovesdy CP, et al: Association between changes in hemoglobin and administered erythropoiesis-stimulating agent and survival in hemodialysis patients. J Am Soc Nephrol 2006;17:1181–1191.
39 Stivelman JC: Refractoriness to recombinant human epoetin (rHuEPO) treatment; in Nissenson AR, Fine RN (eds): Handbook of Dialysis Therapy, ed 4. Philadelphia, Saunders Elsevier, 2008, pp 812–831.
40 National Kidney Foundation: KDOQI clinical practice guidelines and clinical practice recommendations for anemia in chronic kidney disease. Am J Kidney Dis 2006;47:S11–S19.
41 Kilpatrick RD, Critchlow CW, Fishbane S, et al: Greater epoetin-α responsiveness is associated with improved survival in hemodialysis patients. Clin J Am Soc Nephrol 2008;3:1077–1083.
42 Szczech LA, Barnhart HX, Inrig JK, et al: Secondary analysis of the CHOIR trial epoietin-α dose and achieved hemoglobin outcomes. Kidney Int 2008;74:791–798.
43 Tentori F, Blayney MJ, Albert JM, et al: Mortality risk for dialysis patients with different levels of serum calcium, phosphorus, and PTH: the Dialysis Outcomes and Practice Patterns Study (DOPPS). Am J Kidney Dis 2008;52:519–530.
44 Young EW, Albert JM, Satayathum S, et al: Predictors and consequences of altered mineral metabolism: the Dialysis Outcomes and Practice Patterns Study. Kidney Int 2005;67:1179–1187.

Dr. Vincenzo Panichi
Nephrology and Dialysis, Versilia Hospital
Via Aurelia, 335, Lido di Camaiore
IT–55041 Camaiore Lucca (Italy)
Tel. + 39 0584 605 7238, E-Mail vpanichi@usl12.toscana.it

Krick G, Ronco C (eds): On-Line Hemodiafiltration: The Journey and the Vision.
Contrib Nephrol. Basel, Karger, 2011, vol 175, pp 129–140

Overcoming the Limitations of Post-Dilution On-Line Hemodiafiltration: Mixed Dilution Hemodiafiltration

Luciano A. Pedrini[a] · Gerhard Wiesen[b]

[a]Nephrology and Dialysis Department, NephroCare, Bolognini Hospital of Seriate, Seriate, Italy;
[b]Fresenius Medical Care, Department of Research and Development, Bad Homburg, Germany

Abstract

The impact of hemodiafiltration (HDF) on survival is still a topic of under investigation. Most recently, the results of two large prospective trials (the CONTRAST Study and the Turkish HDF Study) did not find any difference in survival between on-line HDF versus low- and high-flux hemodialysis (HD) in the overall dialysis population. However, secondary subgroup analyses of both studies showed a significant reduction in death risk among patients on HDF with high volume exchange, confirming the preliminary observation of the European DOPPS Study. Higher middle molecule removal is definitely attained in high-efficiency HDF compared to high-flux HD, and lower basal β_2-microglobulin levels may result in reduced death risk, as suggested by an analysis of the HEMO Study.

In this scenario, a new modality of hemodiafiltration (HDF), namely mixed dilution HDF (mixed HDF), was conceived in the first years of the 21st century that aimed at maximizing the efficiency of HDF while reducing the shortcomings and risks associated with the traditional pre- and post-dilution infusion modes. Mixed HDF is assisted by a feedback control system which automatically adjusts the total infusion/ultrafiltration rate and the ratio between pre- and post-dilution infusion rates at the maximal filtration fraction (FF) tolerated by the system. This system takes patient and flow conditions, internal pressures and hydraulic membrane permeability, and their complex interactions and changes during the session into account. The TMP/UF profile prevents the development of dangerous hydrostatic pressures within the dialyzer and helps to better preserve membrane permeability. This facilitates a significant increase in solute removal during treatment in a wide molecular range as well as minimal protein leakage.

Preliminary clinical results indicate that mixed HDF could be the most powerful convective strategy, easily adapted to every patient, especially those with high hematocrit, excessive hemoconcentration or failure of their refilling capacity to maintain a sustainable ultrafiltration. Such patients typically have a low tolerance for post-dilution HDF.

Domain of the Mixed HDF Concept

Several prospective studies have provided definite evidence that HDF, as compared to standard and high-flux hemodialysis (HD), promotes enhanced removal of small, middle molecular and some protein-bound compounds and succeeds in reducing their basal levels in the long term [1–6]. The result is a sustained improvement in the uremic toxicity profile, which may help to prevent the progression of (or to ameliorate) some severe uremic complications of chronic dialysis treatment, such as anemia [5, 7], chronic inflammation [8, 9], dyslipidemia [7], hyperphosphatemia and secondary hyperparathyroidism [5, 7, 10], all of which lead to accelerated atherosclerosis in dialysis patients. Significantly lower plasma β_2-microglobulin (β_2M) levels, attained with the use of high-flux membranes [1, 3, 4, 11], have been shown to reduce the incidence of dialysis-related amyloidosis and carpal tunnel syndrome [12, 13] and were associated with reduced all-cause and infection-related mortality in dialysis patients [11, 14].

The impact of HDF on hard clinical end-points is still under investigation. However, the available evidence is suggestive of a benefit of convective treatments, at least in some categories of patients and/or treatment modalities. Observational studies on large patient databases with long-term follow-up have shown a reduced mortality risk of around 35% in patients on on-line HDF compared to patients on low- and high-flux HD [9, 15, 16]. A small Italian, randomized study reported a 55% reduced death risk in patients on hemofiltration (HF) compared to low-flux HD over a 3-year period [17]. In a retrospective analysis of the European Dialysis Outcomes and Practice Patterns Study [18], a significant 35% lower mortality risk was only observed in patients on high-efficiency HDF (volume exchange of 15–25 liters/session) compared to low- and high-flux HD, while no difference was observed between low-efficiency HDF and conventional or high-flux HD.

More recently, the results of two large-database, prospective studies comparing survival in patients on on-line HDF versus low-flux HD, the CONTRAST Study [19], and versus high-flux HD, the Turkish HDF Study [20], did not find any difference in survival in the overall dialysis population after a 3- and 2-year follow-up, respectively. However, secondary subgroup analyses of both studies showed a significant reduction in the risk of death for cardiovascular and overall causes among patients on HDF with high volume exchange of over 20 liters/treatment in the CONTRAST Study and over 17.4 liters/session in the Turkish Study.

Even though secondary analyses of prospective studies entail reduced statistical power, the results obtained with high-efficiency HDF are impressive. Certainly HDF results in higher middle molecule removal than high-flux HD, provided that this technique is performed with high volume exchange. In randomized studies comparing the two strategies, a significant difference in basal β_2M levels only emerged when HDF was performed with a mean filtration volume of 21 liters/session [6], but not with a relatively low volume of 8–12 liters/session [3]. These experiences of the past may attractively link to the results of the CONTRAST and Turkish studies in the light of the relation between B_2-M levels and mortality which was suggested by an analysis of the HEMO Study [11, 14].

Scope of Mixed HDF and Infusion Modalities

In the first years of the 21st century, a new modality of HDF, namely mixed dilution HDF (mixed HDF), was conceived and continuously refined with the aim to maximize the efficiency of the HDF while reducing the shortcomings and risks associated with the traditional pre- and post-dilution infusion modes [21–23].

HDF is the strategy enabling the high hydraulic and solute permeability of high-flux membranes to be most properly exploited, but the modality of substitution fluid infusion influences its performance to a different extent [24]. In the case of post-dilution HDF, the most efficient infusion mode, hemoconcentration, high blood viscosity and resistance to flow (all of which progressively increase during the treatment session) limit the ultrafiltration flow rate (Q_{UF}) and may result in capillaries and dialyzer clotting [25]. Thickening of the secondary protein layer, which is proportional to the filtration pressure, results in a permanent and significant reduction of the membrane permeability. This can compromise the efficiency of the sessions and would require the application of increasingly higher and often unpredictable transmembrane pressure (TMP) gradients to maintain the planned Q_{UF} [22]. However, this is often impossible in the face of the consequences described above, and repeated reduction of the infusion and ultrafiltration rates are necessary to avoid technical and clinical problems – at the price of a decline in convective solute removal.

Pre-dilution HDF ensures better rheological and hydraulic conditions than post-dilution, and the possibility of higher infusion rates, but at the price of reduced efficiency due to dilution of the solute concentrations available for diffusion and convection.

Some years ago, the advent of on-line production of sterile substitution fluid facilitated a broad clinical application of HDF and made the use of large volume exchanges at low cost feasible. However, control systems implemented on available dialysis machines were of little help in counteracting the events described above (especially in post-dilution HDF) so that it was difficult to plan and carry out a session in which efficient and safe operational conditions could be maintained. Thus the concept of mixed HDF was born, targeting maintenance of a constant, maximum infusion/ultrafiltration flow under optimal TMP conditions over the whole treatment time. This was achieved by shifting small amounts of infusion from the post- to the pre-infusion site according to changes in TMP. It was during the realization of the mixed HDF project that a TMP-reactive feedback mechanism was first developed and applied in a clinical setting [22]. This feedback mechanism was able to optimize Q_{UF} and so achieve the most efficient convective transport while maintaining a safe pressure/flow within the dialyzer through the reactive control of TMP. A schematic representation of the mechanism is depicted in figure 1.

Optimization of Sustainable Convection

Several observations form the basis of the new technique, which will be explained in the following.

Maximizing Treatment Efficiency. At a given blood flow, the maximal efficiency in convective solute removal occurs at the highest achievable FF [21], i.e. the ratio between ultrafiltration rate Q_{UF} and plasma water flow rate Q_{PW}. Maximal achievable FF is often unpredictable individually and variable during the treatment due to changing conditions of the membrane permeability, as described above, and to a patient variability, mainly related to the individual refilling capacity as ultrafiltration progresses. At any given blood flow, TMP is exponentially related to the FF, and the slope of the curve is a function of the hydraulic permeability of the dialyzer [21]. Above a certain TMP level, the system enters a critical state and sudden dangerous pressure increases are likely to result from small changes in blood flow or viscosity, venous pressure, or for technical reasons [25]. These events are difficult to prevent or counteract without a feedback system which is able to automatically ensure the highest convective efficiency while maintaining optimal operational conditions in the hemodialyzer. Figure 2 shows how the highest convective removal is achievable theoretically under operational conditions independent of patient and dialyzer parameters.

Conditioning of the Membrane. High-flux membranes, generally having a cutoff up to 60 kDa, may be responsible for massive protein leakage, mainly when high filtration pressure is applied to the intact membrane in the early phase of the session. Even large molecules such as albumin may be forced into the intact pores and either cross them and get lost in the dialysate or be entrapped inside, with the effect of a partial obstruction of the pores and a permanent and

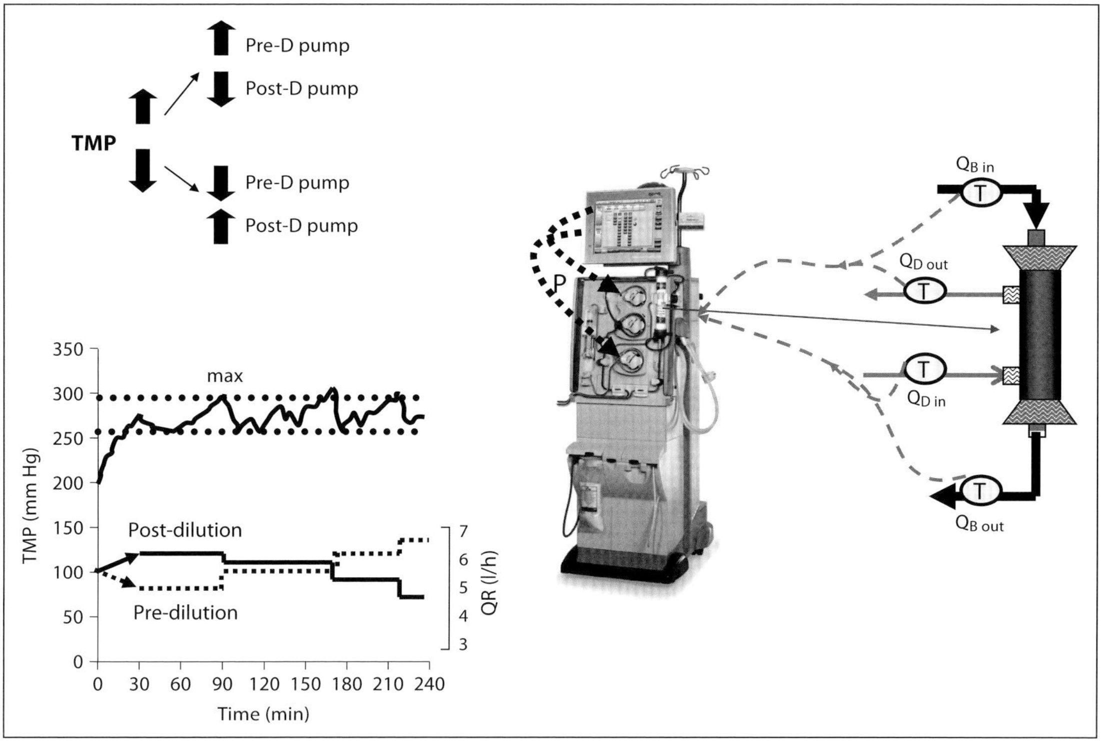

Fig. 1. Schematic representation of on-line mixed HDF with the TMP/Q_{UF} feedback control system. TMP is continuously calculated from measures obtained with four pressure transducers (T) placed at inlet and outlet blood and dialysate ports (right side of the figure). Sterile infusion fluid, prepared on-line with double ultrafiltration, is driven to the infusion ports of the dialyzer by means of two peristaltic pumps (P) at relative infusion rates modulated by the TMP/Q_{UF} feedback through changes of the pumps speed. TMP is forced to follow a definite profile during the session by modulating the ratio between pre- and post-dilution in order to optimize the filtration fraction (left side of the figure).

significant reduction of the membrane permeability. If a low Q_{UF} is set at the start of the session, i.e. less transmembrane driving force, only small peptides and proteins are driven to the membrane surface and adhere more regularly to the inner surface of its pores. Compared to the pristine membrane, this secondary membrane layer shows smaller pore sizes, but permeability to middle molecular solutes like β_2M is not substantially modified, whereas larger plasma molecules, such as albumin, are rejected or integrated into the secondary membrane. Based on these findings, the mixed HDF treatment was designed to start with low filtration pressure at the beginning of the session by setting relatively low FF (0.35–0.40) obtained with a prevailing rate of substitution fluid infused in pre-dilution. Then, with the help of the TMP feedback, TMP is ramped up gradually by means of automatic shifts of small amounts of the infusion fluid

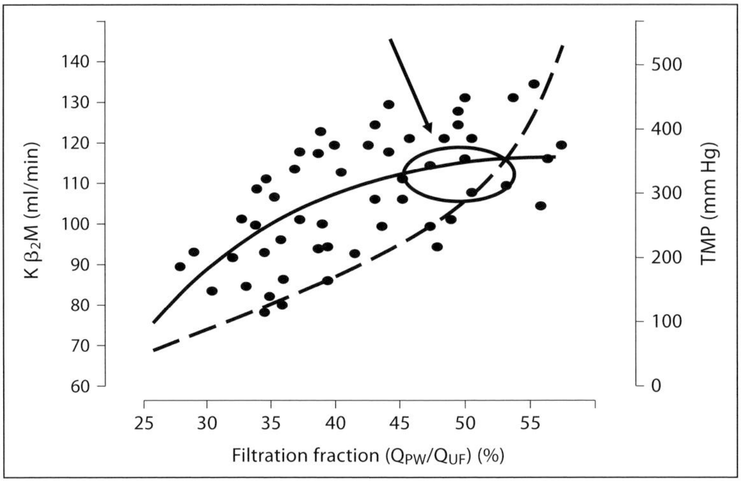

Fig. 2. Relationship between filtration fraction (FF, X-axis), β_2M clearance (K β_2M, left Y-axis) and transmembrane pressure (TMP, right axis) tested in mixed HDF patients K β_2M increases with FF increase up to a FF value of about 50%, where the curve reaches its plateau, depending on the applied blood flow rate (here $Q_B = 400$ ml/min). Beyond these FF values, the exponential TMP curve becomes steeper and it is likely to cause technical and clinical problems. The ellipse in the figure delimits the domain of operational conditions which may ensure maximal efficiency (highest K β_2M) under safe hydraulic and flow conditions.

from pre- to post-dilution until it achieves the defined TMP range without reducing the total Q_{UF}.

Principles and Parameterization of Mixed Dilution HDF

On-line mixed HDF was originally performed in our center on a 4008 H on-line Fresenius system (Fresenius Medical Care, Germany) modified with the application of a Y-shaped infusion line and an additional pump on one Y branch that diverted part of the total infusion from the post-filter to the pre-filter infusion site. A feedback system for TMP control was used in mixed HDF to modulate the pre-dilution/post-dilution ratio while maintaining the total infusion constant throughout the session (fig. 1). The basic concept is that splitting and varying the infusion between pre- and post-filter in order to treat with an optimal relative filtrate flow rate guarantees the best possible rheological and hydraulic conditions within the dialyzer at the highest fluid exchange rate and with maximal solute removal by convection.

The control variable, i.e. the mean pressure gradient between blood and dialysate compartments along the dialyzer (TMP, mm Hg), was calculated on-line by means of a dedicated software analyzing signals from pressure transducers located at the inlet and outlet blood and dialysate ports of the dialyzer ($P_{B\ in}$, $P_{B\ out}$, $P_{D\ in}$, $P_{D\ out}$, respectively) using the equation:

$$TMP = 0.5 \bullet [(P_{B\ in} + P_{B\ out}) - (P_{D\ in} + P_{D\ out})] - P_{onc} \qquad (1)$$

where P_{onc} (mm Hg) is the mean oncotic pressure exerted by the plasma proteins, set by default to a constant value of 25 mm Hg. TMP was kept in a specified TMP window by both adjusting the overall substitution volume and the momentary distribution of pre- and post-dilution flow rates.

As mentioned above, the FF was defined arbitrarily as the fraction of $Q_{PW\ in}$ filtered during the passage through the dialyzer:

$$FF = (1 - Q_{PW\ out}/Q_{PW\ in}) = Q_{UF}/Q_{PW\ in} \qquad (2)$$

where the suffix 'in' and 'out' define flow at the inlet and outlet dialyzer port. $Q_{PW\ in}$ was determined online from the effective blood flow rate ($Q_{B\ eff} = Q_B$ compensated for the arterial pressure in front of the blood pump), from hematocrit (Hct), monitored on-line with an integrated device (blood volume monitor, FMC), and from the water fraction of plasma (F_p), according to the classic equation:

$$Q_{PW\ in} = Q_{B\ eff} \bullet (1 - Hct/100) \bullet F_p \qquad (3)$$

The initial infusion rate (Q_S) was usually set equal to $Q_{PW\ in}$ but, according to the clinical needs of the individual patient and the characteristics of the dialyzer, different values for $Q_S/Q_{PW\ in}$ ratio were chosen between 0.7 and 1. With a lower post-dilution rate at the start of the treatment (FF from 0.3 to 0.5), a slow start with a progressive TMP ramp in the first 30 min could be realized in order to condition the dialyzer membrane.

An optimal patient-specific setting of both initial and treatment FF could be evaluated after 3–6 mixed HDF treatments. Typical values for the overall substitution volume would be up to 50% of the processed blood volume, delivered in close to equal proportions both in pre- and post-dilution. With a new algorithm, the 5008 dialysis machine evaluates and adapts the treatment settings in an automatic way including the data from the last treatment stored for each patient.

Mixed HDF with Closed Loop Control and Adaption Mode

As discussed above, mixed HDF offers the two principal possibilities of choosing the substitution volume relative to blood or plasma water flow and the split of the substitution volume in pre- and post-dilution volumes to maximize the treatment result with respect to convective clearances.

The mixed HDF treatment setting is controlled in two phases. In the initial phase of approximately 15 min an optimal secondary membrane layer formation is primed by inducing progressive small increases in TMP from its initial low values (about 100 mm Hg) up to its preselected range (from 260–280 to 300–330 mm Hg). After this initial TMP ramp, the first closed loop control keeps TMP values within the planned range by preventing excessive increase in TMP with infusion shifts from post- to pre-dilution with the effect to reduce the FF or, vice versa, by compensating for drops in TMP with infusion shifts from pre- to post-dilution that increase the FF. Besides that, TMP can also be stabilized by reducing the total infusion rate in small steps to compensate for the progressive hemoconcentration caused by the weight loss and recorded on-line by means of the BVM. In this mode, fewer shifts between post- and pre-dilution are necessary to maintain constant TMP values.

A second closed loop control algorithm aims at a balanced treatment result in terms of both dilution modalities. High FF values would cause the TMP values to repeatedly exceed the upper limit of the target range and, as a consequence, the treatment would develop towards a pre-dilution HDF treatment. Low FF would drive the treatment in the opposite direction, i.e. would eventually result in a post-dilution treatment. The adaption algorithm varies the FF value in order to keep the treatment result balanced in terms of the volume split before and after the dialyzer. In a first version, the objective was set to equally distributed volumes as this showed the best results for middle molecular clearances [22]. Depending on future clinical results, modified versions could aim at different ratios emphasizing either pre- or post-dilution depending on the specific clearance or anticoagulation and clinical needs of the patient concerned.

Experimental and Clinical Results of Mixed HDF

Continuous improvement of the mixed HDF technique was carried out in the first years of this century following experimental application in selected centers and with a limited number of patients. Since its implementation on the new 5008 Fresenius Dialysis System, several European Dialysis Centers have started to offer this advanced therapy to their patients.

Theoretical validation of the new HDF technique was obtained in an experimental setting [26] by comparing the clearances of different molecular weight dextran fractions measured by means of size exclusion chromatography and obtained during the three HDF infusion modes (mixed, pre- and post-dilution) and during high-flux HD. The curves derived and depicted in figure 3 showed that the clearance in the molecular weight range between 2 and 60 kDa, covered by three different dextran fractions, were always higher for mixed HDF than for the other HDF modalities and HD. The small loss of urea clearance results from the pre-dilution component and corresponding decrease of the diffusion gradient.

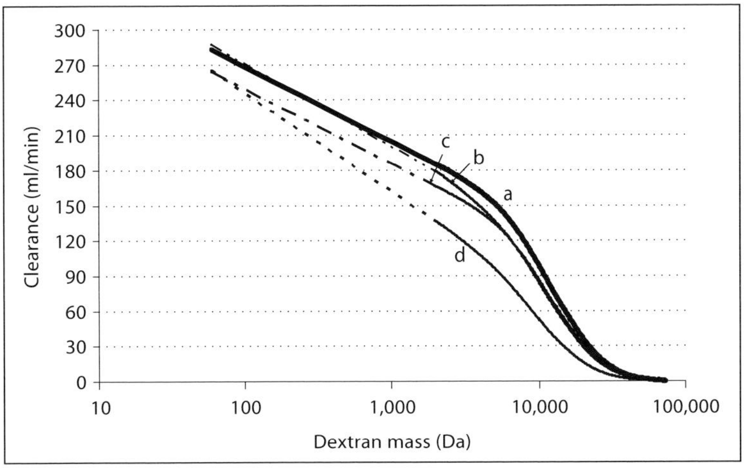

Fig. 3. Dextran clearance comparison between various HDF techniques (a, mixed HDF; b, post-dilution HDF; c, pre-dilution HDF) and high-flux HD (d), performed with a 5008 Dialysis Machine (FMC, Bad Homburg, Germany) and a high-flux dialyzer (FX800, FMC). Clearance was measured by means of size exclusion chromatography (Agilent 1200 System) using a mix of three technical grade dextran fractions with 3.5, 15 and 40 kDa (flow rate 300 ml/min). The clearance curves start at 60 Da with the value of the clearances for urea, which was added to the dextran mix. All components were dissolved in a NaCl solution at a concentration of 0.35 mol/l, the same NaCl solution was used as 'dialysis fluid'. Due to the NaCl artifact in the measurements, all values from 60 to 2,000 Da were replaced by a line between the urea value and the first dextran clearance value of 2,000 Da. From this value on, the curves only represent dextran clearances. All treatment settings corresponded to the default settings of the 5008 Dialysis Machine.

Clinical controlled trials published to date showed that mixed HDF performed at the maximal infusion/ultrafiltration rate possible in post-dilution HDF (FF ~50%) achieved similar efficiency in small solute removal while ensuring safe hydraulic conditions similar to pre-dilution HDF [21]. The advantage of mixed HDF clearly appeared with respect to middle molecule removal when higher infusion rates were applied under the feedback control, which allowed the TMP to be set and modulated according to a defined ultrafiltration profile. Convective transport was optimized under these conditions and on-line mixed HDF yielded a significantly higher β_2M removal than that obtained in pre- and post-dilution [22, 23] (fig. 4) and in mid-dilution HDF [27], a convective technique recently proposed and claimed to be of greater efficiency when compared to the traditional pre- or post-dilution infusion modes in HDF [28]. Different diffusive and convective dialysis modalities were compared in an independent multicenter study recently published [29]. In this study, the highest Kt/V for urea and β_2M were reported in the patients of the mixed HDF group among a total study population of 407 subjects.

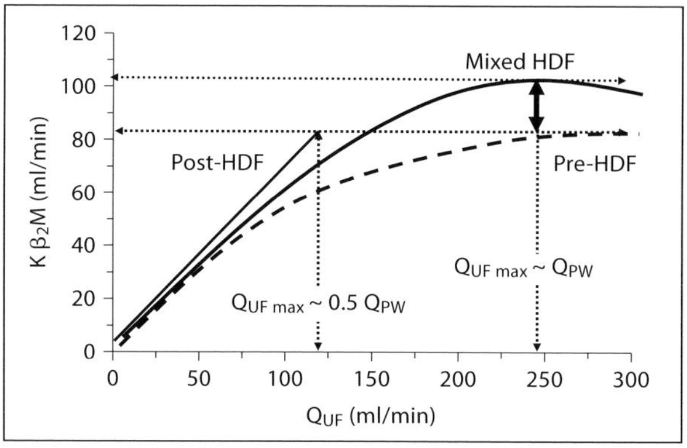

Fig. 4. Relations between ultrafiltration rate (Q_{UF}, X-axis) and β_2M clearance (K β_2M, Y-axis) in on-line HDF with different infusion modalities (blood flow rate, $Q_B = 400$ ml/min, plasma water flow rate, $Q_{PW} = 242$ ml/min). The linear relation is limited in post-dilution by the maximal FF achievable with this infusion mode. The exponential curve for K β_2M in pre-dilution reaches a plateau when the Q_{UF} rate approximates Q_{PW}. This trend is similar in mixed HDF but the K β_2M curve reached its plateau at a higher value. The possible advantage in K β_2M achievable with mixed HDF is shown by the arrow.

Remarkably, superior results in mixed HDF compared to mid-dilution HDF were obtained with the application of much lower pressure regimen within the dialyzer by means of the TMP/Q_{UF} profile, thus better preserving the permeability of the membrane and minimizing the protein leakage favored by very high hydrostatic pressures.

The feedback automatically adjusts the infusion ratio between pre- and post-dilution at the maximum FF without reducing the total infusion and taking into account flow conditions, internal pressures, membrane permeability and their complex interactions and changes occurring during the sessions. For this reason, mixed HDF may be of special advantage in patients with high predialysis hematocrit and an increased risk of filter clotting with post-dilution HDF due to hemoconcentration [30]. Moreover, this new infusion modality may offer the possibility to keep all those patients on HDF therapy who could hardly be submitted to post-dilution HDF due to failure of their refilling capacity and therefore to a scarce availability of ultrafiltrable plasma water (e.g. patients with diabetes, heart failure, autonomic nervous system diseases). In fact, the feedback mechanism efficiently compensates for the progressive hemoconcentration occurring during the treatment by proportional addition of small amounts of pre-dilution infusion fluid to the blood entering the dialyzer.

References

1 Lin CL, Yang CW, Chiang CC, Chang CT, Huang CC: Long-term on-line hemodiafiltration reduces predialysis β_2-microglobulin levels in chronic hemodialysis patients. Blood Purif 2001;19:301–307.

2 Lin CL, Huang CC, Yu CC, Yang HY, Chuang FR, Yang CW: Reduction of advanced glycation end product levels by on-line hemodiafiltration in long-term hemodialysis patients. Am J Kidney Dis 2003;42:524–531.

3 Locatelli F, Mastrangelo F, Redaelli B, Ronco C, Marcelli D, La Greca G, Orlandini G: Effects of different membranes and dialysis technologies on patient treatment tolerance and nutritional parameters. The Italian Cooperative Dialysis Study Group. Kidney Int 1996;50:1293–1302.

4 Pedrini LA, De Cristofaro V, Comelli M, Casino FG, Prencipe M, Baroni A, Campolo G, Manzoni C, Coli L, Ruggiero P, Acquistapace I, Auriemma L: Long-term effects of high-efficiency on-line haemodiafiltration on uraemic toxicity. A multicentre prospective randomized study. Nephrol Dial Transplant 2011;26:2617–2624.

5 Vaslaki L, Major L, Berta K, Karatson A, Misz M, Pethoe F, Ladanyi E, Fodor B, Stein G, Pischetsrieder M, Zima T, Wojke R, Gauly A, Passlick-Deetjen J: On-line haemodiafiltration versus haemodialysis: stable haematocrit with less erythropoietin and improvement of other relevant blood parameters. Blood Purif 2006;24:163–173.

6 Ward RA, Schmidt B, Hullin J, Hillebrand GF, Samtleben W: A comparison of on-line hemodiafiltration and high-flux hemodialysis: a prospective clinical study. J Am Soc Nephrol 2000;11:2344–2350.

7 Pedrini LA, DeCristofaro V, Comelli M, Casino FG, Prencipe M, Baroni A, Campolo G, Manzoni C, Coli L, Ruggiero P, Acquistapace I, Auriemma L: Long-term effects of high-efficiency on-line haemodiafiltration on uraemic toxicity. A multicentre prospective randomized study. Nephrol Dial Transplant 2011;26:2617–2624.

8 Kim HW, Yang HN, Kim MG, Choi HM, Jo SK, Cho WY, Kim HK: Microinflammation in hemodialysis patients is associated with increased CD14CD16+ pro-inflammatory monocytes: possible modification by on-line hemodiafiltration. Blood Purif 2011;31:281–288.

9 Panichi V, Rizza GM, Paoletti S, Bigazzi R, Aloisi M, Barsotti G, Rindi P, Donati G, Antonelli A, Panicucci E, Tripepi G, Tetta C, Palla R: Chronic inflammation and mortality in haemodialysis: effect of different renal replacement therapies. Results from the RISCAVID Study. Nephrol Dial Transplant 2008;23:2337–2343.

10 Minutolo R, Bellizzi V, Cioffi M, Iodice C, Giannattasio P, Andreucci M, Terracciano V, Di Iorio BR, Conte G, De Nicola L: Postdialytic rebound of serum phosphorus: pathogenetic and clinical insights. J Am Soc Nephrol 2002;13:1046–1054.

11 Cheung AK, Rocco MV, Yan G, Leypoldt JK, Levin NW, Greene T, Agodoa L, Bailey J, Beck GJ, Clark W, Levey AS, Ornt DB, Schulman G, Schwab S, Teehan B, Eknoyan G: Serum β_2-microglobulin levels predict mortality in dialysis patients: results of the HEMO Study. J Am Soc Nephrol 2006;17:546–555.

12 Koda Y, Nishi S, Miyazaki S, Haginoshita S, Sakurabayashi T, Suzuki M, Sakai S, Yuasa Y, Hirasawa Y, Nishi T: Switch from conventional to high-flux membrane reduces the risk of carpal tunnel syndrome and mortality of hemodialysis patients. Kidney Int 1997;52:1096–1101.

13 Locatelli F, Marcelli D, Conte F, Limido A, Malberti F, Spotti D: Comparison of mortality in ESRD patients on convective and diffusive extracorporeal treatments. The Registro Lombardo Dialisi e Trapianto. Kidney Int 1999;55:286–293.

14 Cheung AK, Greene T, Leypoldt JK, Yan G, Allon M, Delmez J, Levey AS, Levin NW, Rocco MV, Schulman G, Eknoyan G: Association between serum β_2-microglobulin level and infectious mortality in hemodialysis patients. Clin J Am Soc Nephrol 2008;3:69–77.

15 Vilar E, Fry AC, Wellsted D, Tattersall JE, Greenwood RN, Farrington K: Long-term outcomes in online hemodiafiltration and high-flux hemodialysis: a comparative analysis. Clin J Am Soc Nephrol 2009;4:1944–1953.
16 Jirka T, Cesare S, Di Benedetto A, Perera CM, Ponce P, Richards N, Tetta C, Vaslaky L: Mortality risk for patients receiving hemodiafiltration versus hemodialysis. Kidney Int 2006;70:1524–1525.
17 Santoro A, Mancini E, Bolzani R, Boggi R, Cagnoli L, Francioso A, Fusaroli M, Piazza V, Rapana R, Strippoli GF: The effect of online high-flux hemofiltration versus low-flux hemodialysis on mortality in chronic kidney failure: a small randomized controlled trial. Am J Kidney Dis 2008;52:507–518.
18 Canaud B, Bragg-Gresham JL, Marshall MR, Desmeules S, Gillespie BW, Depner T, Klassen P, Port FK: Mortality risk for patients receiving hemodiafiltration versus hemodialysis: European results from the DOPPS. Kidney Int 2006;69:2087–2093.
19 Grooteman M, van den Dorpel R, Bots M, Penne L, van der Weerd N, Mazairac A, den Hoedt C, van der Tweel I, Levesque R, Nubé M, ter Wee P, Blankestijn P: Online hemodiafiltration versus low-flux hemodialysis: effects on all-cause mortality and cardiovascular events in a randomized controlled trial. The Convective Transport Study (CONTRAST). 2011 (in press).
20 Ok E, Asci G, Ok ES, Kircelli F, Yilmaz M, Hur E, Demirci MS, Ozdogan O, Demirci C, Sertoz OO, Duman S, Ozkahya M, Kaykcioglu M, Elbi H, Basci A, Toz H: Comparison of postdilution on-line hemodiafiltration and hemodialysis (Turkish HDF Study). 2011 (in press).
21 Pedrini LA, De Cristofaro V, Pagliari B, Sama F: Mixed predilution and postdilution online hemodiafiltration compared with the traditional infusion modes. Kidney Int 2000;58:2155–2165.
22 Pedrini LA, DeCristofaro V: On-line mixed hemodiafiltration with a feedback for ultrafiltration control: effect on middle-molecule removal. Kidney Int 2003;64:1505–1513.
23 Pedrini LA, Cozzi G, Faranna P, Mercieri A, Ruggiero P, Zerbi S, Feliciani A, Riva A: Transmembrane pressure modulation in high-volume mixed hemodiafiltration to optimize efficiency and minimize protein loss. Kidney Int 2006;69:573–579.
24 Pedrini LA: On-line hemodiafiltration: technique and efficiency. J Nephrol 2003;16(suppl 7):S57–S63.
25 Henderson LW: Biophysics of ultrafiltration and hemofiltration; in Maher JF, (ed): Replacement of Renal Function by Dialysis. Dordrecht, Kluwer Academic, 1989, pp 300–326.
26 Sharifi H, Wiesen G, Vienken J, Mottaghy K: Analysis of low- to middle-molecular clearance ratios in haemodialysis and different haemofiltration dilution options using a method based on dextrans and size exclusion chromatography; Master Thesis in Biomedical Engineering, RWTH, Aachen, Germany 2010.
27 Feliciani A, Riva MA, Zerbi S, Ruggiero P, Plati AR, Cozzi G, Pedrini LA: New strategies in haemodiafiltration (HDF): prospective comparative analysis between on-line mixed HDF and mid-dilution HDF. Nephrol Dial Transplant 2007;22:1672–1679.
28 Krieter DH, Collins G, Summerton J, Spence E, Moragues HL, Canaud B: Mid-dilution on-line haemodiafiltration in a standard dialyser configuration. Nephrol Dial Transplant 2005;20:155–160.
29 Casino FG, Pedrini LA, Santoro A, Mandolfo S, David S, De C, V, Teatini U, Lomonte C, Lopez T: A simple approach for assessing equilibrated Kt/V β_2M on a routine basis. Nephrol Dial Transplant 2010;25:3038–3044.
30 Kuhlmann MK: Phosphate elimination in modalities of hemodialysis and peritoneal dialysis. Blood Purif 2010;29:137–144.

Dr. Luciano A. Pedrini
U.O. Nefrologia e Dialisi, NephroCare, Ospedale Bolognini
Via Paderno 21, IT–24068 Seriate/BG (Italy)
Tel. +39 035 306 3259
E-Mail luciano.pedrini@fmc-ag.com

Krick G, Ronco C (eds): On-Line Hemodiafiltration: The Journey and the Vision.
Contrib Nephrol. Basel, Karger, 2011, vol 175, pp 141–151

Fifteen Years of Experience with On-Line Hemodiafiltration

Francisco Maduell

Department of Nephrology, Hospital Clinic Barcelona, Barcelona, Spain

Abstract

Hemodiafiltration (HDF) with elevated substitution fluid offers an optimal way of removing uremic substances. The beginnings of HDF and on-line HDF, learning curve, differences in the removal of uremic toxins, difficulties in the development, automated manual Q_i as a practical way of prescribing, distinct experiences with on-line HDF and prospective, randomized ongoing on-line HDF studies are detailed as a personal vision for 15 years' handling with on-line HDF.

Hemodialysis ensures the survival of close to 2 million patients with chronic renal failure worldwide. After more than four decades of chronic dialysis treatment, the level of technological development is satisfactory and hemodialysis can be considered a routine renal replacement therapy with guaranteed short-term safety. The long-term clinical outcome, however, could be improved. Malnutrition is common, hyperphosphatemia, hypertension and heart failure control is poor, rehabilitation and quality of life are suboptimal, and hospitalization and mortality rates are high. Cardiovascular disease is the most common cause of mortality in chronic hemodialysis patients and is the reported cause of death in approximately 50%. Depner defined this situation as a residual syndrome that includes susceptibility to infection, reduced maximal oxygen consumption during exercise, sleep disturbances, depression, impaired mental concentration, reduced stamina and markedly increased susceptibility to cardiovascular complications.

Beginnings of Hemodiafiltration

In the 1990s, there were several priorities in the field of hemodialysis. The first aim was to reduce dialysis time to 3.0–3.5 h per session in order to improve patient quality of life. This required increased solute removal during the session using increases in blood flow (Q_b), dialysate flow (Q_d) and dialyzers with a larger surface area (1.6–2.1 m^2). Technological advances in dialysis machines, especially volumetric control of ultrafiltration and the widespread use of bicarbonate in the dialysis fluid, allowed the use and development of synthetic dialyzers with larger pores and high hydraulic permeability. Thus, blood depuration of higher molecular weight substances could be achieved. These membranes heralded a new era in hemodialysis and opened new fields of study and treatment, namely high-flux hemodialysis and convective techniques such as hemofiltration and hemodiafiltration (HDF). Initially, given the design of dialysis machines, simple HDF techniques were used that involved off-line production of replacement fluid. The initial experience gained with HDF techniques was used in Spain to shorten the length of the dialysis sessions. HDF increased efficacy and tolerance of treatment, and the high quality of the dialysis fluid/substitution fluid used avoided the type of back-filtration-induced adverse reactions reported when high-flux membranes were first introduced. Exogenous replacement fluid was necessary but was limited to <10 liters per session for practical reasons (infusion replacement was limited by the dialysis machine to 2 l/h; 4 l/h when a precision balance was used) and financial considerations (exogenous solutions are expensive). These HDF techniques included biofiltration, conventional HDF, paired filtration dialysis and acetate-free biofiltration. High-flux hemodialysis is a form of low-volume HDF because of the internal filtration and back-filtration that can take place within a dialyzer. Although quantification of back-filtration is still controversial, flow rates were estimated by Dr. Claudio Ronco et al. to be up to 30 ml/min, and may generate 4–8 liters of back-filtration in a 4-hour session. Clinical experience has confirmed that there are no differences between high-flux dialysis and low-volume HDF.

During the 1990s, nephrologists were aware that water treatment was adequate but still did not meet the requirements for water for ultrapure dialysis fluid. Consequently, the entry of dialysis fluid into the blood compartment (called back-filtration) was avoided as much as possible. Acute symptoms were listed as pyrogenic reactions, hypoxia and hypotension, while chronic symptoms were understood to be chronic inflammation, increased susceptibility to infections, amyloidosis, malnutrition and arteriosclerosis.

Beginnings of On-Line Hemodiafiltration

To perform HDF with large volumes of replacement fluid, a feasible technique for preparing cheap, clean substitution fluid is required. Many approaches have been employed to test and ensure the microbiological quality of the water used for dialysis or dialysate. These technical innovations have enabled on-line production of ultrapure substitution fluids in large quantities for high-efficiency HDF procedures. After Henderson successfully produced sterile, pyrogen-free solutions by ultrafiltration in 1978, several new HDF techniques appeared with large-volume, on-line preparation of replacement fluid for HDF. These new HDF techniques included high-flux HDF and on-line HDF.

High-Flux HDF. Von Albertini achieved very high clearances for both small and large solutes using two large high-flux dialyzers in series and adjusting the pressures over the filters so that ultrafiltration occurs only in the first filter and back-filtration only in the second filter. Ultrafiltration in the first device was 116 ml/min and the total filtrate removed per 2-hour treatment session averaged 13 liters. One member of this research group, Dr. Juan Bosch, was invited to a symposium on 'Advances in Hemodialysis' in Burgos, Spain, in 2004, to speak about this experience. His presentation taught me personally that, if pure water and ultrapure dialysate are available, back-filtration can become an effective ally in achieving better solute removal.

Dialysis machines have been modified to perform on-line HDF. This technique involves adding one or two filters at intermediate points in the dialysate line to produce clean dialysate, and an infusion pump to divert a specific fraction of the dialysate produced (50–200 ml/min or 3–12 l/h). The total infusion volume is limited only by the blood flow (one-third of blood flow) and the transmembrane pressure (TMP), which is determined by the ultrafiltration, hematocrit, total proteins and session length. With blood flow rates of 350–450 ml/min and infusion rates of 100–130 ml/min, over 24–32 liters of convective transport is provided during a 4-hour treatment session. Dr. Bernard Canaud showed that on-line HDF is a safe, well-tolerated technique and good clinical results have been observed with the first prototype dialysis machines in Europe.

In Spain, the first experiences date back to 1993, in Granada, where Dr. Juan Garcia-Valdecasas, who had previously visited von Albertini's group, was interested in highly convective techniques and reinfusion dialysis fluid and had the opportunity to work with on-line HDF prototype machines with satisfactory results. I was very interested in these techniques and followed these initial experiences with great interest. Then, in September 1996, I had the opportunity to work with the first machines marketed for on-line HDF.

Working with high-volume HDF techniques was highly gratifying because they offer several advantages over conventional low-flux or high-flux hemodialysis methods, as well as over low-volume HDF techniques. First, the use of high-permeability synthetic membranes, which provide the best biocompatibility, is required. Second, HDF with high volumes of replacement fluid is an optimal way of removing uremic substances over a wide range of molecular sizes, from small solutes to low-molecular-weight proteins. Third, performance of these techniques requires the use of ultrapure dialysate, which provides other benefits for the patient [1–9].

Patients' opinions and their degree of satisfaction with clinical and laboratory findings quickly confirmed that we were on the right road. Furthermore, as in most groups, we discontinued short dialysis and switched to three times weekly sessions of a minimum of 4 h each.

Learning Curve in On-Line Hemodiafiltration

Blood Flow

In on-line HDF, the most important limiting factor for the infusion rate (Q_i) is the blood flow (Q_b) and TMP [10]. Machines for post-dilution HDF allow an infusion rate of 30% of Q_b, so this is the approach we took in the beginning. Later, with the experience gained, we concluded that a Q_i of 25% or less of Q_b is preferable in order to avoid increasing the blood viscosity and causing clotting complications within the circuit. These complications trigger numerous machine alarms that affect the normal operation of a treatment session for both the patient and the medical staff. To optimize the use of post-dilutional HDF, we recommend a Q_b of between 360 and 500 ml/min with a Q_i of between 80 and 125 ml/min.

Dialyzers

We were also curious to examine whether the choice of dialyzer for on-line HDF is important [11]. In a study of eleven different dialyzers, only triacetate and PMMA (polymethylmethacrylate) were found to be of limited use for conducting on-line HDF, basically because of TMP-related problems. The other dialyzers evaluated (i.e. polysulfone and derivatives, polyamide, polyacrylonitrile, AN69 and PEPA) could perform on-line HDF without problems at similar TMPs controlled by the dialysis machines.

Vascular Access

Initially an arteriovenous fistula was considered the best and only option for on-line HDF. However, the use of catheters has increased in recent years (between 15 and 20% of patients on hemodialysis). Because of the aging population and increased prevalence of vascular disease, tunneled catheters were reconsidered in on-line HDF patients. In 1998, Canaud et al. published 7 cases of permanent catheters in on-line HDF and Maduell et al. reported 8 cases of on-line HDF in patients with tunneled catheters and a Q_b of 372 ml/min with a mean infusion volume of 20.1 ± 4 liters (between 18 and 25 liters).

Pre-Dilutional, Post-Dilutional or Mixed Infusion

After a review of the literature and our own studies, we believe that post-dilutional infusion is the most effective form of infusion for the removal of all substances (small, medium and large molecules) – even if part of the circuit may be susceptible to technical problems because of hemoconcentration and increased TMP. Pre-dilutional infusion prevents some such technical problems but reduces the clearance of solutes due to dilution of their concentrations. Mid-dilution is a recent alternative with infusion taking place in the middle of the dialyzer, whereby infusion is post-dilution HDF for the first half of the dialyzer and pre-dilution HDF for the second half. This provides similar or even superior results to the post-dilution mode [12, 13]. We still await the practical application and results of mixed dilution HDF, which is characterized by simultaneous pre- and post-dilution and autoregulation of both flows. This could optimize efficacy and avoid hemoconcentration.

Differences between Hemodialysis and On-Line Hemodiafiltration Regarding Removal of Uremic Toxins

Solute removal is the primary goal of dialysis and, as 50,000 Da is the cut-off of the natural kidney, substances up to this molecular weight should ideally be removed. Different solute clearance profiles are obtained depending on the treatment mode selected. HDF with high volumes of replacement fluid seems to be the most effective technique for removing all small, medium-sized and large molecules. Low-flux hemodialysis only removes solutes with molecular weights of less than 5,000 Da. Several studies have analyzed the removal capacity of different treatment modes over a broad spectrum of solutes. Urea and creatinine clearances largely depend on diffusion processes. Small solutes (<500 Da) are effectively removed by all treatment modes except hemofiltration. β_2-Microglobulin (11,800 Da) is not removed by low-flux hemodialysis because this molecule is larger than the membrane pore size. Thus its clearance is largely achieved by high-flux dialysis and convection processes. Kerr et al., Lornoy et al. and Maduell et al. have reported a reduction rate for β_2-microglobulin of 50–60% in high-flux hemodialysis and of 70–80% in on-line HDF.

Our group was also very interested in the removal of solutes of molecular weight exceeding that of β_2-microglobulin [14–16]. The use of high-volume convection techniques plays an important role in the removal of solutes larger than 15,000 Da during hemodialysis. Like β_2-microglobulin, however, these larger molecules have a low distribution volume and/or follow a multicompartmental model as reflected by the difficulties of normalizing predialysis plasma concentrations. Healthy kidneys work 24 h a day to maintain normal levels of uremic toxins. The results of our studies suggest that the removal of solutes larger than β_2-microglobulin, such as myoglobin, prolactin and α_1-microglobulin, is difficult with high-flux therapies so that highly convective treatment could possibly be applied. Other studies support this hypothesis: Lepenies et al. observed that the extraction ratio for leptin was higher with convective techniques, and Ward et al. studied complement factor D and found that its removal was significantly higher for on-line HDF than for high-flux hemodialysis.

Difficulties in the Development of On-Line Hemodiafiltration

The expansion of convective techniques to becoming routine treatment has been delayed for technological and economic reasons. Hemofiltration or HDF modalities require the use of high-permeability dialyzers and, at the same time, machines with volume control and a dual pump. Replacement fluid constitutes a further cost factor: this was the main reason for abandoning hemofiltration (replacement volumes exceed 20 liters), and was a key constraint in the initial HDF technique with volumes ranging between 3 and 10 liters. Finally, the introduction of on-line HDF techniques using the dialysis fluid itself as a replacement solution has required major changes to be made to hemodialysis units. It has taken another 10 years to refurbish and upgrade water treatment systems, acquire specific machines and incorporate safety filters to ensure a high quality of this replacement fluid (ultrapure dialysate).

The availability of excellent water treatment systems and ultrapure dialysate has led to a breakthrough in the clinical treatment of patients on dialysis and represents the first major achievement of on-line HDF. Nevertheless, on-line HDF was only used in less than 10% of patients in 2000. Another essential requirement for routine use of on-line HDF is tests for endotoxin determination, which often had to be referred to outside laboratories.

'Automated Manual Q_i' Is a Practical Way of Prescribing Post-Dilution On-Line Hemodiafiltration

The most commonly used mode of infusion is post-dilution on-line HDF, since it provides high clearance of small and large solutes although it can cause a greater number of complications related to hemoconcentration and TMP. While the pre-dilution mode partially solves such technical problems, it also reduces the efficiency of solute removal because of hemodilution. Hemodialysis research is currently aimed at obtaining safer, more practical and effective systems, which largely depend on technical advances to improve dialysis machines. Specifically, to adjust the replacement rate of a manual post-dilution on-line HDF treatment, the recommended Q_i is 25% of Q_b. Some of these machines (Fresenius 5008) offer the possibility to automatically adjust Q_i with a formula using real values for total protein and hematocrit. Furthermore, the ultrafiltration coefficient is measured in the first few minutes of the dialysis session and subsequently every hour. Additional measurements are performed if any unexpected events occur. The cyclic pressure test is performed, which estimates and monitors (by means of TMP) the behavior of the dialyzer curve during treatment, progressively adjusting Q_i.

If we decide to graduate Q_i manually, the machine will not modify Q_i automatically and we have to modify this value when we detect an alarm or warning on the machine resulting from TMP increases. Indeed automatic Q_i modification may not even be feasible if hematocrit and total protein values are not known (one does not always have the results of analysis for each session), as these are required for the formula. In such a case, one can use 'automated manual' or 'alarm-free' treatment. Here we prescribe a Q_i value automatically by adjusting hematocrit and total protein values to obtain a Q_i value for manual prescription at the beginning of the session.

In a study performed in 2007, our group showed that automated manual Q_i prescription in post-dilution on-line HDF is able to meet the treatment prescription (normally a Q_i of about 25% of the Q_b) with an individual intradialysis adaptation according to blood viscosity and hemoconcentration [17]. We concluded that prescription of automated manual Q_i is a practical way of prescribing post-dilution on-line HDF in which maximum efficacy and total replacement volume are achieved with a significant reduction in the number of alarms during dialysis. This, consequently, improves the patients' clinical course without delaying the end-time.

Distinct Experiences with On-Line Hemodiafiltration

Daily On-Line HDF

In September 2001, our group decided to combine the most physiological and effective dialysis schedule (daily dialysis) with on-line HDF [18, 19]. Patients on standard 4- to 5-hour three times weekly on-line HDF were switched to 2- to 2.5-hour six times weekly on-line HDF. Although the dialysis time was similar in both treatment schedules, an increase in the dialysis dose was obtained with the daily scheme, confirming the beneficial effect of the higher frequency. The principal advantages observed in this study were excellent clinical tolerance and patient acceptance, disappearance of post-dialysis fatigue, improvement of sleep disorders, higher removal of middle and large molecules with a 21% reduction in predialysis plasma β_2-microglobulin levels, a reduction in phosphate binders, improvement of nutritional status (body weight increased from 67.8 ± 8 to 69.4 ± 8 kg after 6 months and to 70.9 ± 9 kg after 1 year), better control of blood pressure without antihypertensive medication and regression of left ventricular hypertrophy.

Nocturnal, In-Center, Every-Other-Day On-Line HDF

In 2007, we began a new phase in Hospital Clinic in Barcelona when we sought to combine the most physiological and effective dialysis schedule, long (nocturnal) and more frequent (every-other-day) dialysis with the dialysis modality that offers the highest solute and uremic toxin removal (on-line HDF). The aim of this study was to switch patients from standard 4- to 5-hour three times weekly on-line HDF to 7–8 h sessions every other day with on-line HDF [20].

We observed that this change produced excellent clinical tolerance and patient acceptance, adequate social and occupational rehabilitation, better dialysis adequacy, remarkable improvement in nutritional status, regression of left ventricular hypertrophy, and good phosphate and hypertension control with a substantial reduction in the need for phosphate binders and antihypertensive medication.

Prospective, Randomized Ongoing On-Line Hemodiafiltration Studies

The year 2007 was instrumental in the development of on-line HDF in Catalonia since this treatment modality was promoted by the local government: the Catalonian Health Authorities gave an additional reimbursement for on-line HDF to dialysis care providers. The Catalonian Society of Nephrology promoted a prospective, randomized, open study to evaluate the potential benefits regarding patient survival of on-line HDF over standard hemodialysis: the '*Estudio de Supervivencia de Hemodiafiltración On-Line*' (ESHOL)'. This is an ongoing study that has enrolled 906 patients, 50% on high-flux hemodialysis and 50% on on-line HDF with post-dilutional infusion, with a follow-up period of 3 years [21]. The primary objective is survival. As the coordinator of this study, I had the opportunity to teach on-line HDF to more than 20 hospitals and dialysis centers through theoretical and practical sessions in 2007 and 2008. It was very rewarding to share our experience and interact with a large number of colleagues and nursing staff to assist in the implementation of this technique and help dispel any doubts that arose.

There are also several other ongoing multicenter, prospective randomized studies that may help to determine whether convective techniques are superior to hemodialysis or not. However, each of these studies has a different design (table 1).

An Italian multicenter study has enrolled 146 patients, of which 50% receive low-flux HD, 25% receive on-line HDF with pre-dilutional infusion, and 25% receive pre-dilutional hemofiltration. The follow-up is 2 years.

The Dutch Convective Transport Study (CONTRAST) aims to include 800 patients, 50% on low-flux HD, and 50% on post-dilutional on-line HDF. The monitoring period is 3 years and the primary objective is survival.

A French multicenter study aims to include 600 patients over 65 years of age, 50% on high-flux hemodialysis and 50% on post-dilutional on-line HDF. The monitoring period is 2 years and the primary goal is intradialytic tolerance.

Table 1. Some ongoing studies comparing on-line HDF and HD

	Italian study	French study	Contrast study	Turkish HDF study	ESHOL study
Country	Italy	France	Netherlands	Turkey	Catalonia, Spain
Design	RCT	RCT	RCT	RCT	RCT
Number	146	420	700	780	906
Baseline year	2004	2005	2004	2007	2007
Final year of study	2008	2010	2010	2010	2011
Groups compared	Pre-dilution HDF-OL/HF vs. low-flux HD 1:1:2	Post-dilution HDF-OL vs. high-flux HD 1: 1	Post-dilution HDF-OL vs. low-flux HD 1:1	Post-dilution HDF-OL vs. high-flux HD 1:1	Post-dilution HDF-OL vs. high-flux HD 1:1
Primary endpoint	Cardiovascular tolerance and blood pressure	Intradialytic tolerance	Mortality	Mortality and cardiovascular events	Mortality
Outcome	2 years	2 years	3 years	2 years	3 years

HD = Hemodialysis; HDF = hemodiafiltration; HF = hemofiltration; OL = on-line; RCT = randomized controlled trial.

A Turkish study aims to include 800 patients, 50% on high-flux hemodialysis and 50% on post-dilutional on-line HDF. The monitoring period is 2 years and the primary purpose is to evaluate cardiovascular morbidity and mortality.

Conclusions

In view of reports in the literature and our own experience, now is the time to switch to convective techniques [22]. Firstly, because technological development in water treatment and advances in dialysis machines, as well as the widespread use of synthetic high-flux dialyzers, make this a feasible proposition. Indeed, the latest generation of dialysis machines, known as therapeutic systems, are designed to work under convective conditions at all times using the dialysis fluid itself as the replacement solution. Secondly, we have listed the possible clinical benefits of these treatments and have found no published literature reporting any undesirable effects. We eagerly await receiving further scientific evidence from the ongoing multicenter studies.

References

1 Maduell F, del Pozo C, García H, Sánchez L, Hdez-Jaras J, Albero MD, Calvo C, Torregrosa I, Navarro V: Cambio de hemodiafiltración convencional a hemodiafiltración en línea. Seguimiento un año. Nefrología 1998;18:308–315.

2 Maduell F, del Pozo C, García H, Sánchez L, Hdez-Jaras J, Albero MD, Calvo C, Torregrosa I, Navarro V: Change from conventional haemodiafiltration to on-line haemodiafiltration. Nephrol Dial Transpl 1999; 14:1202–1207.

3 Maduell F, Puchades MJ, Navarro V, Rius A, Torregrosa E, Sánchez JJ: Valoración de la medición de la dosis de diálisis con dialisancia iónica en hemodiafiltración on-line. Nefrología 2005;25:521–526.

4 Maduell F: Hemodiafiltration. Hemodial Int 2005;9:47–55.

5 Maduell F, Navarro V: Bases of cardiovascular and hematological effects. Hemodial Int 2006;10:S38–S41.

6 Alcazar R, Maduell F, Marti A: Reconocimiento de las distintas modalidades de hemodiálisis. Nefrología 2006;26(suppl 8): 22–33.

7 Maduell F: Optimizing the prescription of hemodiafiltration. Contrib Nephrol. Basel, Karger, 2007, vol 158, pp 225–231.

8 Maduell F, Arias A: Indicaciones y prescripción de la hemodiafiltración. Dial Traspl 2008;29:62–66.

9 Maduell F, Navarro V, Hdez-Jaras J, García H: Sangrias de repetición a un paciente en hemodiálisis. Nefrología 1998;18:339–340.

10 Maduell F, García H, Hdez-Jaras J, Calvo C, Navarro V: Depuración de solutos en hemodiafiltración en línea. Influencia del flujo de sangre y de infusión. Nefrología 1999;19:28–35.

11 Maduell F, Navarro V, Hdez-Jaras J, Calvo C: Comparación de dializadores en hemodiafiltración en línea. Nefrología 2000;20:269–276.

12 Maduell F, Arias M, Vera M, Fontseré N, Blasco M, Barros X, Garro J, Elena M, Bergadá E, Cases A, Bedini J, Campistol JM Mid-dilution hemodiafiltration: a comparison with pre- and post-dilution mode using the same polyphenylene membrane. Blood Purif 2009;28:268–274.

13 Maduell F, Arias M, Fontseré N, Vera M, Mass E, Garro J, Barros X, Martina MN, Elena M, Bergadá E, Cases A, Bedini JL, Campistol JM: What infusion flow should be used for mid-dilution hemodiafiltration? Blood Purif 2010;30:25–33.

14 Maduell F, Navarro V, Cruz MC, Torregrosa E, Garcia D, Simon V, Ferrero JA: Osteocalcin and myoglobin removal in online hemodiafiltration versus low and highflux hemodialysis. Am J Kidney Dis 2002;40: 582–589.

15 Maduell F: Eficacia depurativa de medianas y grandes moléculas en diferentes modalidades de hemodiálisis. Nefrología 2005;25(suppl 2): 15–18.

16 Maduell F, Sánchez–Canel JJ, Blasco JA, Navarro V, Rius A, Torregrosa E, Pin MT, Cruz MC, Ferrero JA: Depuración de grandes moléculas. Más allá de la β_2-microglobulina. Nefrología 2006;26:469–475.

17 Maduell F, Arias M, Garro J, Vera M, Fontseré N, Barros X, Massó E, Martina MN, Sentis A, Duran C, Bergadá E, Cases A, Campistol JM: Pauta de infusión manual automatizada: una forma práctica de prescribir la hemodiafiltración on-line automatizada. Nefrología 2010;30:349–353.

18 Maduell F, Navarro V, Torregrosa E, Rius A, Dicenta F, Cruz MC, Ferrero JA: Change from thrice weekly on-line hemodiafiltration to short daily on-line hemodiafiltration. Kidney Int 2003;64:305–313.

19 Maduell F, Navarro V, Rius A, Torregrosa E, Sánchez JJ, Saborit ML, Ferrero JA: Mejoría del estado nutricional con hemodiafiltración en línea diaria. Nefrología 2004;24:60–66.

20 Maduell F, Arias M, Durán C, Vera M, Fontseré N, Azqueta M, Massó E, Martina MN, Pérez N, Sentis A, Elena M, Bergadá E, Cases A, Bedini JL, Campistol JM: Nocturnal, every-other-day, on-line hemodiafiltration: an effective therapeutic alternative. Nephrol Dial Transpl 2011 (E-pub ahead of print).

21 Maduell F, Moreso F, Pons M, Ramos R, Mora J, Forester A, Soler J, Galceran JM, Martinez-Castelao A, on behalf of the On-Line Hemodiafiltration Study Group from the Catalonian Society of Nephrology: Design and patient characteristics of ESHOL study: Postdilution on-line haemodiafiltration versus haemodialysis, a Catalonian prospective randomised study. J Nephrol 2011; 24:196–202.

22 Maduell F: Controversias en Hemodiálisis: Convección versus Difusión. ¿Ha llegado el momento del cambio? Nefrología 2009;29:613–617.

Francisco Maduell
Department of Nephrology, Hospital Clínic Barcelona
Villarroel, 170
ES–08036 Barcelona (Spain)
Tel. +34 932275447, E-Mail fmaduell@clinic.ub.es

Krick G, Ronco C (eds): On-Line Hemodiafiltration: The Journey and the Vision.
Contrib Nephrol. Basel, Karger, 2011, vol 175, pp 152–162

Adopting On-Line Hemodiafiltration as Standard Therapy in EMEA NephroCare Centers

Andrea Stopper · Laura Scatizzi · Gerdi Klinkner · Carlo Boccato · Aileen Grassmann · Daniele Marcelli

Fresenius Medical Care, NephroCare Coordination, Bad Homburg, Germany

Abstract

This paper describes the historical journey that led to the adoption of on-line hemodiafiltration (HDF) as a standard therapy for the patients in the Fresenius Medical Care (FME) NephroCare dialysis network. In 1998, FME faced the tremendous challenge of consolidating a series of heterogeneous clinics under one umbrella. In 2002, the European Best Practice Guidelines (EBPG) for hemodialysis (HD) were published by the European Renal Association which FME promptly adopted within its clinic network. On the basis of this document, the strategic decision was taken to apply high-flux, biocompatible membranes throughout the entire network. To cope with the effective implementation of this step, the clinics' technical infrastructure was updated. The widespread application of high-flux therapy, together with the implementation of the required infrastructure, especially concerning water quality, opened the way to the extensive use of on-line HDF. To fully realize this ambitious goal, two further technological steps were targeted and successfully reached: introduction of the Fresenius 5008 dialysis equipment and an even stricter control of the water quality. The combined pressure from the educational activities, which brought about a preliminary cultural change, and the creation of a target based on the percentage of treatments by this technique resulted in an increasing implementation of this modality by the individual clinics. After 2004, on-line HDF continuously increased its share among the dialysis techniques prescribed in the network and currently more than 50% of patients are on this modality.

When in 1996 the dialysis division of Fresenius, then a product company, merged with National Medical Care, the leading dialysis service provider in the USA, Fresenius Medical Care (FME) was created. Thereafter, FME became a

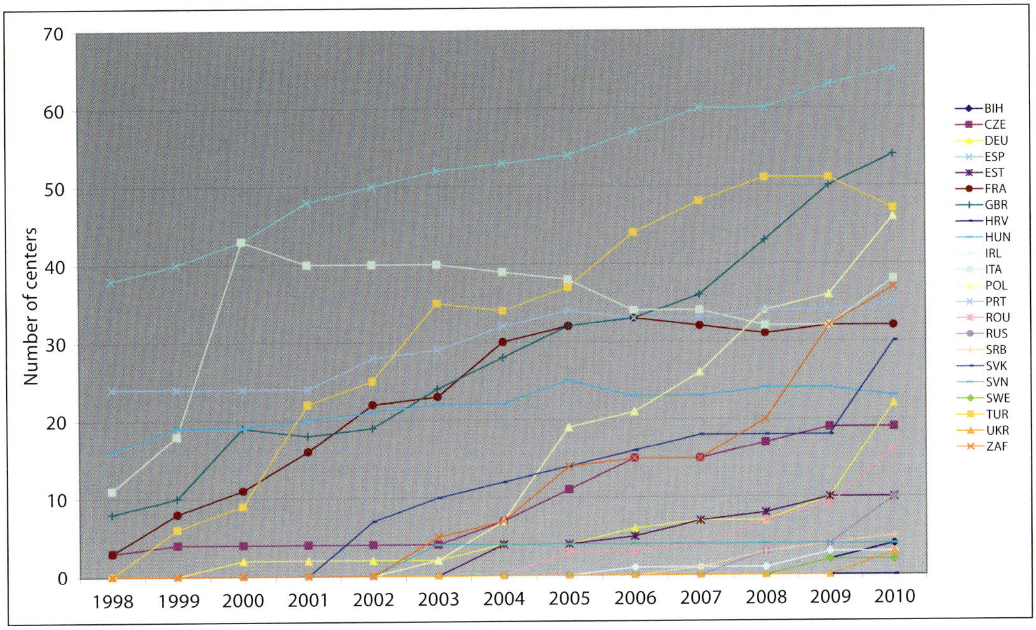

Fig. 1. Development of dialysis centers in the NephroCare EMEA Network from 1998 to 2010.

world player in the provision of dialysis services. In Europe, the new company started dialysis service activity with a group of about 100 National Medical Care clinics that were principally located in Portugal and Spain. Ever since then, FME has been expanding its presence in Europe and beyond, quickly creating a major global dialysis network through new acquisitions, construction of de novo clinics, clinic privatization and participation in public tenders [1] (fig. 1). Currently, the FME dialysis network of the region Europe, Middle East and Africa (EMEA) – nowadays represented by name NephroCare – comprises over 550 clinics in 23 countries, and treats more than 44,000 patients.

This paper describes the historical journey of FME that led to the adoption of on-line hemodiafiltration (HDF) as a standard therapy for the patients in its NephroCare network.

Setting Standards

Naturally, the move to becoming a global dialysis provider resulted in a change of focus for FME. It was obvious from the beginning of this new activity that the company's vision had to be adapted to recognize the significance of the patient in his/her central role as being the most valuable asset [1]. This meant a fundamental change in company philosophy from a product-centric organization to a patient-centric one. This realization led to a new mission that is still valid today: ensuring all patients in all clinics of the network the delivery of dialysis treatments that result in the best clinical outcome possible, while continuously improving the patients' quality of life.

Up to the merger, the non-US based clinics were managed directly from the headquarters of National Medical Care. After the merger, FME faced the tremendous challenge of consolidating a series of heterogeneous clinics under one umbrella. The diversity between the clinics in terms of treatment modalities, quality of service and technical infrastructure soon made an organizational split between the US domestic market and the market of EMEA necessary. Most of these inter-facility differences originated from the beliefs and convictions of the original founders of the individually acquired units and from challenging constraints, mainly of economical nature, of the national and even local healthcare systems. One example is the practice of dialyzer reuse, which was still common in Portugal at the time of the merger. Consequently, a dedicated department was created in Europe to meet these challenges – Clinical Management Europe (CME).

CME started its activities in 1998 and was responsible for the coordination of all activities in the steadily growing network from a clinical point of view and for the entire EMEA region. This responsibility ranged from clinical governance to technical coordination as well as the allocation of training resources and provision of guidance from a corporate perspective. After having stopped the reuse practice in all NephroCare clinics, the next milestone was to organize the collection of patient data in each center in order to facilitate analysis of treatment modalities and evaluation of outcomes. This was initially done by manual monthly data collection via Excel sheets where information about numbers of prevalent patients, patient movements, changes of treatment, outcomes, etc. were collected and reported. The data collection would not have been possible without the tremendous support from the staff in the centers. In the following step, FME developed a specific clinical database in 1999 called EuCliD (European Clinical Database) to collage the key medical information on the treatment of dialysis patients [2]. EuCliD soon became an essential component of the Continuous Quality Improvement program of FME. It is a multi-lingual and fully codified software applying international standard coding tables (ICD 10, ISCED, national pharmaceutical data bases, etc.) and contains sensitive patient medical data while simultaneously ensuring strict data confidentiality.

In 1993, the first clinical guideline in the field of dialysis was issued by the US Renal Physicians Association [3]. The Dialysis Outcomes Quality Initiative (DOQI) guidelines followed in 1997 [4–7]. Following the American example, several European national bodies – for example, the European Dialysis and Transplantation Association (EDTA) [8], the British Renal Association [9], and the Società Italiana di Nefrologia [10] – prepared their own guidelines adapted to European or national conditions. However, it soon became obvious that the mere availability of guidelines was not sufficient to ensure quality. Guidelines needed to be implemented and their application continuously monitored in order to guarantee that a high quality of care is delivered to the patients. In 2002, the European Best Practice Guidelines (EBPG) for hemodialysis (HD) were published by the European Renal Association [11]. Subsequently, FME decided to officially adopt this set of guidelines within its clinic network.

The implementation of Clinical Practice Guidelines was accompanied by the rolling out of supporting programs, namely the Clinical Performance Measures, the Patients' Safety Initiatives and the Continuous Quality Improvement programs. All of these initiatives in the network took advantage of the previously developed computerized monitoring system EuCliD [12]. In fact, since the beginning, EuCliD allowed the verification of the success of all quality-related activities within the FME dialysis clinics by comparison of the results with internal and external benchmarks.

Focus on High-Flux Dialysis

FME aimed, on the basis of the EBPG, to create a common strategic treatment platform targeting improved patient outcomes in terms of quality of life and survival.

Consequently, on the basis of EBPG sections III.1 and III.2, the strategic decision was taken to adopt high-flux, biocompatible membranes throughout the entire network.

EBPG III.1: *'Dialyzer membranes with the lowest degree complement and leukocyte activation should be applied. Dialyzer membranes that induce strong complement and leukocyte activation, inflammatory reactions, and/or a blunting of the response of leukocytes to stimuli should be avoided'*;

EBPG III.2: *'To achieve an improved clinical outcome regarding morbidity and mortality, the use of large pore/high-flux biocompatible dialyzers should be preferred'*.

To facilitate realization of this first Quality Implementation Measure, a preparatory step was identified as necessary: updating of the clinics' technical infrastructure to cope with the effective implementation of high-flux dialysis. One of these aspects was related to the chemical and, in particular, biological quality of the dialysis water.

The network then proceeded to undertake a multitude of exertions to create and maintain a technical and organizational infrastructure that ensures that all necessary instruments and methods are properly implemented. The instruments to be adopted for these therapies were mainly based on: (a) proper control of dialysis fluid quality, achieved mainly through correct design and implementation of the water treatment system and careful quality control of the produced fluids; (b) dialysis machines equipped with the most up-to-date technology including the dialysis fluid filter, DIASAFE® Plus; and (c) use of high-

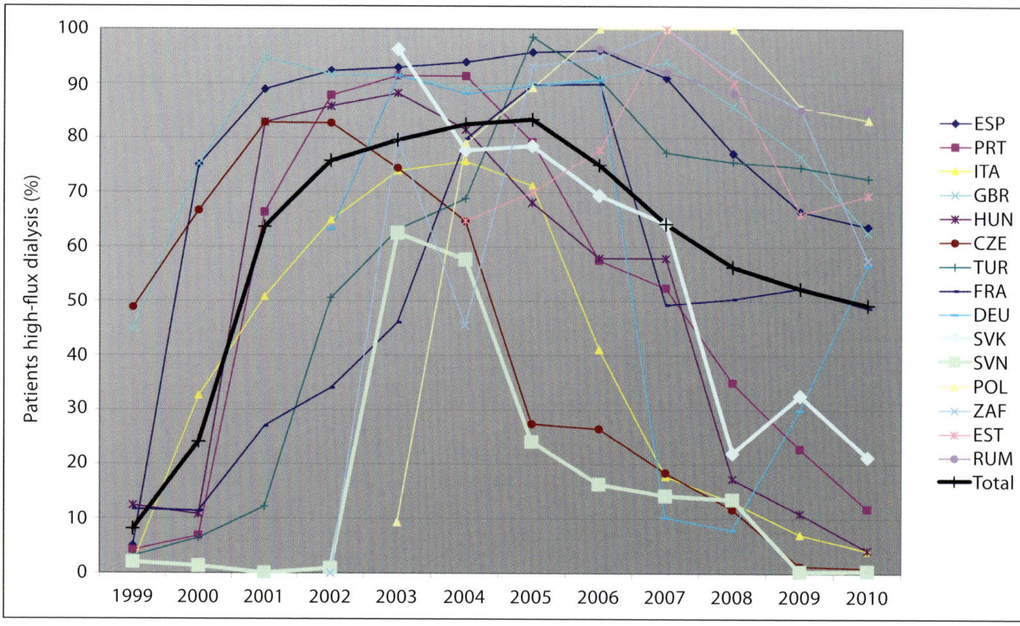

Fig. 2. Proportion of patients on high-flux dialysis in the NephroCare EMEA Network from 1999 to 2010.

flux polysulfone filters. The above aspects also required considerable efforts in terms of operator training. During these years, the company organized training sessions for all involved personnel to enable them to deal effectively with all new technical and medical issues.

The successful implementation of the EBPG was certified on the basis of the evidence collected with EuCliD [13]. As reported in figure 2, at the time of EuCliD implementation (1999), only 8.1% of patients were treated with high-flux dialysis. The public review of the draft of the EBPG on HD involving the international nephrological community (e.g. EDTA congresses, etc.) created a strong focus on the advantages of high-flux dialysis. Therefore, not surprisingly, even prior to the official issue of the guideline a spontaneous increase of the application of high-flux dialysis, wherever possible, was observed. The publication of the EBPG in 2002 boosted this development further. The preliminary promising results were validated by an internal study published by Merello Godino et al. [14] showing an improvement in the field of anemia correction, a decreased level of β_2-microglobulin and an improved lipid metabolism. By 2003, more than 80% of patients had been moved to this advantageous technology. The MPO study finally confirmed in 2009 this modality to be superior to low-flux [15]. The NephroCare network participated directly in this European trial with a number of centers in Portugal and France. At that time the major concern in relation to the use of high porosity membranes was related to safety aspects. It has to be underlined that, even prior to the MPO publication, the NephroCare experience, which is based on millions of high-flux dialysis treatments, demonstrated the absolute safety of the technique.

Driving Change Forward

In the meantime, in parallel with the implementation of these new measures relating not only to high-flux dialyzers but also to dialysis fluid quality and dialysis machine technology, the network continued to expand the number of centers in the original group and in additional countries. What emerged was the need to combine clinical governance with the management of all other network aspects (e.g. technical) in a continuously changing environment. The new approach to patient care, which was based on simultaneous integration of the perspectives of all stakeholders (patients, employees, shareholders, community) and a holistic therapy concept, eventually merged under the NephroCare umbrella. This approach embraces the complete philosophy of care delivered to the patients ranging from dialysis products to therapies including renal pharmaceuticals (all of which are constantly being improved), as well as care from qualified, motivated clinic personnel who regularly receive further training.

The NephroCare Balanced Scorecard is the primary methodology used to reach this goal. This tool is applied to optimize patient outcome by interrelating key performance indicators addressing medical (patient) and financial aspects (shareholders) as well as internal (employees) and environmental (community) processes.

On-Line HDF as Standard Therapy

HDF combines diffusion and convection in order to facilitate the removal of high and low molecular weight solutes and has been shown to be superior to all other treatment modalities currently available. However, possible pyrogenic reactions pose a considerable threat to the patients since the risk of microbiological contamination is increased. Besides, costs are higher with increasing volumes of substitution fluid used. Therefore, the availability of high purity substitution fluid at lower cost was a clear requirement for the broad application of the modality.

In this regard, the widespread application of high-flux therapy, together with the implementation of the required infrastructure, especially concerning water quality, opened the way to the extensive use of on-line HDF therapy. This step was also recommended in sections II.2.1 and II.2.2 of the EBPG:

EBPG II.2.1: *'β2-m is representative in its kinetic behaviour of other MM and peptides of similar size, and may be used as a marker for such molecules'.*

EBPG II.2.2: '*To enhance MM removal, synthetic high-flux membranes should be used. Additional strategies, such as adding a convective component, or increasing HD time or frequency, should be used to maximize MM removal*'.

The financial constraints were largely resolved with the technique of 'on-line' fluid production resulting in the availability of unlimited volumes of ultra-pure substitution fluid at a cost close to that of dialysate for conventional HD [16, 17].

To fully realize the goal of establishing on-line HDF as a standard therapy, two further technological steps were targeted and successfully reached: introduction of the Fresenius 5008 therapy system and an even stricter control of the water quality. The latter was achieved by the creation of a company-internal guideline for dialysis fluids. The guideline was implemented in accordance with recognized international regulations (e.g. European Pharmacopoeia and ISO standards) and with the setting up of a dedicated data collection system integrated in EuCliD. In fact, FME played an important role in the review of the ISO standards: the experience collected in the network through the large number of HDF treatments already performed constituted a major contribution to this review. The result was the introduction of technically consistent regulations for the safe and sustainable implementation of on-line HDF.

However, these regulations were in themselves still not sufficient to guarantee highest treatment quality and safety: attention must also be paid to the design and organization of the dialysis center as they have a major impact on work efficiency and on the ability of the personnel to comply with essential rules, such as hygiene. Accordingly, in addition to the above-mentioned guideline on water and dialysis fluids, other internal guidelines were developed. These related to the centers' architectural design, to hygiene and nursing processes.

Moving from high-flux dialysis to on-line HDF was considered a major step also from a cultural viewpoint. To prepare the clinical staff for this major change, on-line HDF was included as an official topic in the accreditation meetings organized during the years 2005/2006 in the countries of the network. The corresponding topics discussed in these meetings referred to the required purity of water and the rationale for the use of the modality. Having as target the change from standard dialysis to on-line HDF, a detailed and open discussion on risks and benefits of this technique was hosted. The main clinical benefits expected from on-line HDF treatments include hemodynamic stability [18, 19], possibly improved quality of life [20] and a delay in the development of dialysis-related amyloidosis [21]. Survival is also expected to improve [22]. The Dialysis Outcome and Practice Patterns Study (DOPPS), a prospective survey, showed better survival of patients on high efficiency HDF [23].

The combined pressure from the educational activities, which brought about a preliminary cultural change, and the creation of a target based on the percentage of treatments by this technique resulted in an increasing implementation of the modality by the individual clinics.

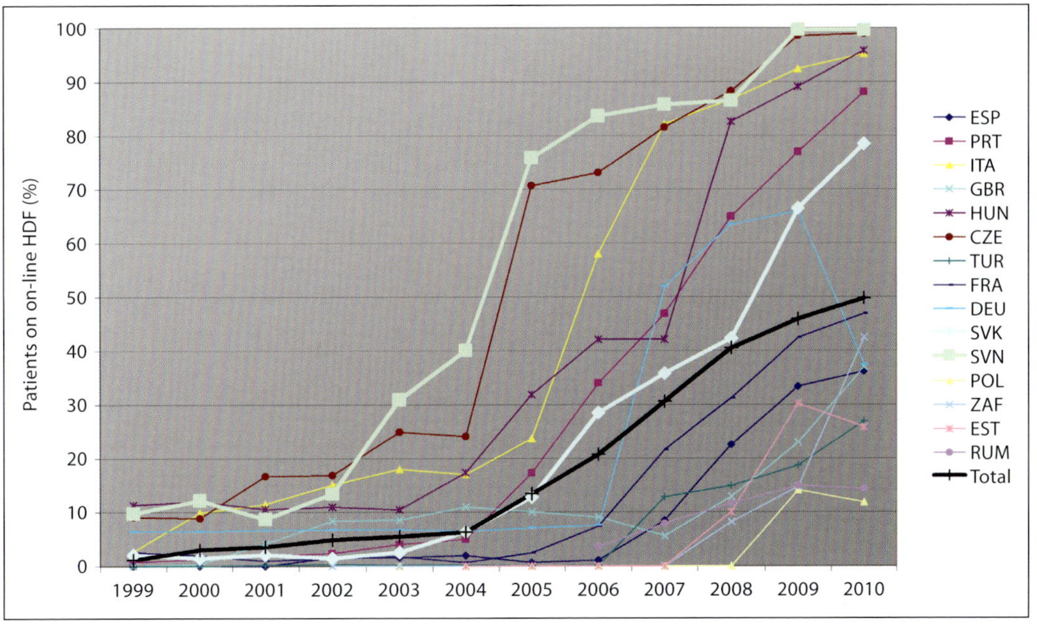

Fig. 3. Proportion of patients on on-line HDF in the NephroCare EMEA Network from 1999 to 2010.

As shown in figure 3, up to 2004, the use of on-line HDF in the NephroCare clinics was rather limited in general. After 2004, on-line HDF increased its share continuously among the dialysis techniques prescribed in the network and currently more than 50% of patients are on this modality. Conversely, the proportion of patients treated with conventional high-flux dialysis progressively decreased after 2005 (fig. 2).

With the progression of the consolidation of the network, the original EuCliD software developed in 1999 fell short of fulfilling the extended documentation requirements associated with on-line HDF. A new version aimed to collect more detailed data on each single dialysis treatment was subsequently developed and implemented in the network. The new project EuCliD 5 was initiated in 2005 and aims to support not only quality assurance, but also the day-to-day work of the clinical staff in all the clinics of the network.

At present NephroCare is addressing two new challenges in its implementation of on-line HDF as standard therapy. The first is a major revision of clinical targets defined in the NephroCare Balanced Scorecard to incorporate new and emerging medical insights. In particular, focus is moving from the per se deployment of on-line HDF to the absolute correctness in the way in which the prescription is carried out. Evidence available in the literature [23] shows that a minimum of 15 liters of reinfusion must be delivered in order to achieve the maximum benefit of on-line HDF for the patient. Consequently, this target has to be achieved in all dialysis sessions and prescription indicators have been replaced by results-related indicators in the NephroCare Balanced Scorecard. The second major challenge is related to the global economic crisis which evolved in 2009. Focus is strong on the achievement of maximum treatment advantage also from an economic point of view. This is reflected in the latest reimbursement models being introduced in countries like Portugal or the US, namely capitation. Capitation is a prospective payment system in which the dialysis treatment providers receive a fixed, predetermined amount of money per capita (capitation) upfront to cover specified services for a defined time period [24, 25]. NephroCare's adoption of on-line HDF as standard therapy serves also to meet the expectation of generating economical savings by decreasing the contribution of pharmaceuticals to the total treatment cost.

In summary, this chapter describes the path of FME, and in particular NephroCare, over the past 13 years, which witnessed the growth from a collection of minor clinic acquisitions to a consolidated and fully integrated dialysis services network ensuring high-quality and cost-efficient treatments, such as on-line HDF, as standard therapy.

Appendix

Country Abbreviations

BIH	Bosnia and Herzegovina
CZE	Czech Republic
ESP	Spain
EST	Estonia
DEU	Germany
FRA	Spain
GBR	Great Britain
HRV	Croatia
HUN	Hungary
IRL	Ireland
ITA	Italy
POL	Poland
PRT	Portugal
ROU	Romania
RUS	Russian Federation
SRB	Serbia
SVK	Slovakia
SVN	Slovenia
SWE	Sweden
TUR	Turkey
UKR	Ukraine
ZAF	South Africa

References

1. Stopper A, Amato C, Gioberge S, Giordana G, Marcelli D, Gatti E: Managing complexity at dialysis service centers across Europe. Blood Purif 2007;25:77–89.
2. Marcelli D, Kirchgessner J, Amato C, Steil H, Mitteregger A, Moscardo V, Carioni C, Orlandini G, Gatti E: EuCliD (European Clinical Database): a database comparing different realities. J Nephrol 2001;14(suppl 4):S94–S100.
3. Renal Physician Association Working Committee on Clinical Practice Guidelines. Washington 1993.
4. NKF-DOQI Clinical Practice Guidelines for Hemodialysis Adequacy. New York, National Kidney Foundation, 1997.
5. NKF-DOQI Clinical Practice Guidelines for Peritoneal Dialysis Adequacy. New York, National Kidney Foundation, 1997.
6. NKF-DOQI Clinical Practice Guidelines for the Treatment of Anemia of Chronic Renal Failure. New York, National Kidney Foundation, 1997.
7. NKF-DOQI Clinical Practice Guidelines for Vascular Access. New York, National Kidney Foundation, 1997.
8. European Best Practice Guidelines for the Management of Anemia in Patients with Chronic Renal Failure. Nephrol Dial Transplant 1999;14(suppl 5):S1–S50.
9. The Renal Association: Treatment of adults and children with renal failure. Standard and audit measures, ed 3, 2002.
10. Gruppi di lavoro delle linee guida SIN: Linee guida della Società italiana di Nefrologia (http://www.sin-italy.org/Governo_Clinico/index.asp), 2003.
11. European Best Practice Guidelines for Hemodialysis (Part 1). Nephrol Dial Transplant 2002;17(suppl 7):S1–S111.
12. Marcelli D, Moscardo V, Steil H, Day M, Kirchgessner J, Mitteregger A, Orlandini G, Gatti E: Data management and quality assurance for dialysis network. Contrib Nephrol. Basel, Karger, 2002, vol 137, pp 293–299.
13. Richards N, Ayala JA, Cesare S, Chazot C, Di BA, Gassia JP, Merello JI, Rentero R, Scatizzi L, Marcelli D: Assessment of quality guidelines implementation using a continuous quality improvement programme. Blood Purif 2007;25:221–228.
14. Merello Godino JI, Rentero R, Orlandini G, Marcelli D, Ronco C: Results from EuCliD (European Clinical Dialysis Database): impact of shifting treatment modality. Int J Artif Organs 2002;25:1049–1060.
15. Locatelli F, Martin-Malo A, Hannedouche T, Loureiro A, Papadimitriou M, Wizemann V, Jacobson SH, Czekalski S, Ronco C, Vanholder R: Effect of membrane permeability on survival of hemodialysis patients. J Am Soc Nephrol 2009;20:645–654.
16. Ledebo I: On-line hemodiafiltration: technique and therapy. Adv Ren Replace Ther 1999;6:195–208.
17. Ledebo I: On-line preparation of solutions for dialysis: practical aspects versus safety and regulations. J Am Soc Nephrol 2002;13(suppl 1):S78–S83.
18. Donauer J, Schweiger C, Rumberger B, Krumme B, Bohler J: Reduction of hypotensive side effects during online haemodiafiltration and low temperature haemodialysis. Nephrol Dial Transplant 2003;18:1616–1622.
19. Locatelli F, Altieri P, Andrulli S, Bolasco P, Sau G, Pedrini LA, Basile C, David S, Feriani M, Montagna G, Di Iorio BR, Memoli B, Cravero R, Battaglia G, Zoccali C: Hemofiltration and hemodiafiltration reduce intradialytic hypotension in ESRD. J Am Soc Nephrol 2010;21:1798–1807.
20. Beerenhout CH, Luik AJ, Jeuken-Mertens SG, Bekers O, Menheere P, Hover L, Klaassen L, van der Sande FM, Cheriex EC, Meert N, Leunissen KM, Kooman JP: Pre-dilution on-line haemofiltration vs. low-flux haemodialysis: a randomized prospective study. Nephrol Dial Transplant 2005;20:1155–1163.
21. Cheung AK, Rocco MV, Yan G, Leypoldt JK, Levin NW, Greene T, Agodoa L, Bailey J, Beck GJ, Clark W, Levey AS, Ornt DB, Schulman G, Schwab S, Teehan B, Eknoyan G: Serum β_2-microglobulin levels predict mortality in dialysis patients: results of the HEMO study. J Am Soc Nephrol 2006;17:546–555.

22 Vilar E, Fry AC, Wellsted D, Tattersall JE, Greenwood RN, Farrington K: Long-term outcomes in online hemodiafiltration and high-flux hemodialysis: a comparative analysis. Clin J Am Soc Nephrol 2009;4:1944–1953.
23 Canaud B, Bragg-Gresham JL, Marshall MR, Desmeules S, Gillespie BW, Depner T, Klassen P, Port FK: Mortality risk for patients receiving hemodiafiltration versus hemodialysis: European results from the DOPPS. Kidney Int 2006;69:2087–2093.
24 Iezzoni LI, Ayanian JZ, Bates DW, Burstin HR: Paying more fairly for Medicare capitated care. N Engl J Med 1998;339:1933–1938.
25 Hackbarth G, Reischauer R, Mutti A: Collective accountability for medical care – toward bundled Medicare payments. N Engl J Med 2008;359:3–5.

Laura Scatizzi
Fresenius Medical Care Deutschland GmbH
NephroCare Coordination EMEA
Else-Kröner-Strasse 1, DE–61352 Bad Homburg (Germany)
Tel. +49 6172 609 5115, E-Mail laura.scatizzi@fmc-ag.com

Krick G, Ronco C (eds): On-Line Hemodiafiltration: The Journey and the Vision.
Contrib Nephrol. Basel, Karger, 2011, vol 175, pp 163–169

Utilization of Hemodiafiltration as Treatment Modality in Renal Replacement Therapy for End-Stage Renal Disease Patients – A Global Perspective

Jan-Michael Sichart · Stefan Moeller

Fresenius Medical Care Deutschland GmbH, Bad Homburg, Germany

Abstract

The worldwide demand for renal replacement therapy (RRT) is constantly rising. In order to support both medical communities and healthcare authorities in their decision-making processes, it has become increasingly interesting to provide quantitative overviews on the global development of the number of end-stage renal disease (ESRD) patients, as well as information on the quantitative development of individual treatment modalities. Worldwide, numerous registries and studies contribute to establishing a reliable base for understanding ESRD patient numbers. Supplementary, Fresenius Medical Care maintains an ESRD information system that enables reporting of the most recent numbers on a global scale. The Fresenius Medical Care Market & Competitor Survey (MCS) provides ESRD-related data from more than 140 countries on a yearly basis. With a combined population of around 6.7 billion, these countries represented around 97% of the world population and covered more than 99% of all treated ESRD patients at the end of 2010. The survey results can be interpreted as providing a global picture of ESRD demographics in 2010, including the number and distribution of patients on individual treatment modalities such as hemodiafiltration (HDF). The following HDF-related results are presented here: the global HDF patient population treated, the HDF patient distribution in various regions/countries, and the growth patterns of HDF and on-line HDF. The treatment of ESRD patients by HDF has gained significantly in popularity over recent years. In some regions, more patients are treated by HDF than by peritoneal dialysis and, in selected countries, HDF accounts for more than 25% of all extracorporeal dialysis treatments for ESRD patients.

End-stage renal disease (ESRD) is a chronic condition with the need for life-saving medical intervention in the form of dialysis or renal transplantation. Worldwide, the size of the prevalent ESRD population is constantly increasing – since the beginning of maintenance therapy for ESRD in the 1960s the number of patients treated for terminal kidney failure has continued to significantly exceed the growth rate of the general population. Consequently, the worldwide demand for renal replacement therapy (RRT) is set to rise and ESRD is increasingly considered an emerging public health problem that requires attention in the medical field as well as in health policy. Therefore, it becomes increasingly interesting to provide quantitative overviews on the global development of ESRD patients as well as information on the quantitative development of individual treatment modalities.

A growing number of national and international renal registries worldwide provide demographic and epidemiologic information on renal patients. The US Renal Data System (USRDS) [1], the multinational European database organized by the ERA/EDTA [2] or the Australia & New Zealand Dialysis and Transplant Registry [3] – to name only a few – contribute to establishing reliable and consolidated information on ESRD patient demographics. An alternative approach to reporting international ESRD-relevant data is pursued in the Dialysis Outcomes and Practice Patterns Study (DOPPS) [4]. These registries and studies constitute an important and well-established base for understanding ESRD treatment practices and policies. However, even at a national level, the maintenance of an information system that enables fast and reliable reporting of the most recent renal patient numbers is particularly challenging. The collection of records reflecting the situation in a large group of countries means a further enhancement of this difficulty. A time lag between data gathering and publication through the registries is inevitable and can be significant at times. Furthermore, national or regional registry data alone cannot offer a complete global picture as the majority of countries providing RRT either do not have official registries or do not publish the corresponding data. (Based on internal Fresenius Medical Care analysis, in 2011 the number of countries publishing information either directly through a national renal registry or indirectly through a multinational organization was 37 while 147 countries are reported to provide renal replacement therapy.) Fresenius Medical Care, the largest dialysis care company worldwide, operating on a global scale, maintains an annually updated database addressing international ESRD data. Through its worldwide network, Fresenius Medical Care is in a unique position to efficiently retrieve and process global ESRD-related information, such as an insight into patient demographics, various aspects associated with the regional patient distribution, treatment practices and trends.

Methods

Details of the data collection and validation process of the Fresenius Medical Care Market & Competitor Survey (MCS) have been described in earlier publications referring to the status in the years 2001, 2004 and 2005 [5–7]. The MCS provides annual data from more than 140 countries (or areas of special sovereignty) with established dialysis programs. With a combined population of around 6.7 billion, these countries represented around 97% of the world population and were estimated to cover more than 99% of all treated ESRD patients at the end of 2010. As such, the survey results can be interpreted as providing a global picture of ESRD demographics in the corresponding year.

The country-by-country survey, consisting of a catalogue of several thematic areas relevant to the treatment of ESRD patients, focuses on the total number of patients treated, the modality selected, trends in treatment practices and products used, treatment location, ESRD patient care structures and funding. Whereas the degree of detail concerning the information requested on ESRD patients and treatment practices varies among different countries depending on maturity and size of their national ESRD patient care program and infrastructure, the modular design of the survey allows the global consolidation and compilation of the gained information in one central database. Before being entered in the database, the surveyed demographic and economic data are additionally validated by means of cross-reference with the most recent sources of national ESRD information (e.g. registry data) and with the results of earlier such surveys performed during previous years. In addition, the collected data are subjected to comprehensive consistency tests. The regular ex-post validations of the survey demonstrate a consecutively high reliability of the acquired data and a systematic bias can be excluded.

In the following, focus is primarily on ESRD patient-related figures at year-end 2010. Results are presented for the subgroup of patients undergoing hemodiafiltration (HDF). The numbers presented are rounded in a consistent and common sense manner.

Results

The utilization of HDF as a treatment modality is quite diverse between the various regions worldwide. Comparing the ratio of HDF patients in a region to the total number of ESRD patients treated by extracorporeal dialysis (here denominated as HD for hemodialysis), Europe is the most relevant HDF region in the world with a share of 15%. Furthermore, Europe also accounts for over 60% of the global HDF population. While the region Asia-Pacific (AP) has a 5% share of its HD patients treated with HDF, the treatment modality is almost non-existent in African, Middle East, Latin and North American countries (table 1).

In terms of absolute numbers, China has become the country with the highest HDF population (13,000 patients), followed by Japan and Germany (each around 10,000 patients).

With 90%, the vast majority of HDF patients receive on-line HDF as defined by the on-line preparation of the substitution fluid by the dialysis machine.

Table 1. Distribution of HD and HDF patients in 2010

	HD patients, n	HD patients on HDF, n	HD patients on HDF, %	HDF patients on conventional HDF, %	HDF patients on on-line HDF, %
Europe total	390,000	57,000	15	5	95
Africa + Middle East + Latin America	330,000	2,000	1	0	100
North America	420,000	300	0	0	100
AP total	680,000	31,000	5	15	85
Global	1,810,000	90,000	5	10	90

Table 2. Distribution of HDF patients in the top ten European countries with largest relative HDF populations in 2010

Country	HD patients n	Patients on HDF total, n	Patients on HDF %
Switzerland	3,000	2,000	>60
Slovenia	1,400	900	>60
Slovakia	2,900	1,600	>50
Portugal	9,900	4,800	>40
Hungary	5,500	2,300	>40
Czech Republic	5,300	1,800	>30
Belgium	6,800	2,000	>30
Greece	8,900	2,600	>25
Sweden	2,900	800	>25
Austria	4,000	1,100	>25

Conventional HDF, as defined by the delivery of substitution fluid from bags, accounted only for 10% of global HDF treatments in 2010.

There were more than 45 countries within the region Europe/Middle East/Africa (EMEA) where HDF treatments were performed in 2010. Table 2 lists the key HDF countries, i.e. those countries where HDF patients account for more than 25% of all HD patients. Switzerland and Slovenia have the highest relative utilization of HDF worldwide, treating more than 60% of all their HD patients with HDF.

It is interesting to see that some of the countries have registered significant increases in HDF utilization over the last years. Between 2004 and 2010, the share of HDF patients increased in Switzerland from ~40% to over 60%, in

Table 3. Distribution of conventional and on-line HDF patients in the top ten European countries with largest HDF populations in 2010

Country	Patients on HDF total n	Patients on conventional HDF %	Patients on on-line HDF %
Germany	9,800		100
Italy	7,600	25	75
France	4,900		100
Portugal	4,800		100
Spain	3,900	5	95
United Kingdom	3,400		100
Greece	2,600	50	50
Hungary	2,300		100
Belgium	2,000		100
Switzerland	2,000		100

Table 4. Growth of HDF patients from 2004 to 2010

HDF patients	2004	2005	2006	2007	2008	2009	2010	CAGR 04-07	CAGR 07-10	CAGR 04-10
Global total	44,000	47,000	50,000	59,000	66,000	77,000	90,000	11%	15%	13%
EMEA total	25,000	27,000	29,000	36,000	43,000	50,000	59,000	13%	18%	15%
Asia-Pacific total	19,000	20,000	21,000	23,000	22,000	27,000	31,000	5%	11%	8%

Slovenia from more than 20% to over 60%, and in Hungary from around 10% to over 40%.

With regard to the absolute numbers of HDF patients in the EMEA region, Germany and Italy are the countries with the largest HDF patient populations (table 3).

What becomes obvious is that, within the top ten EMEA countries with the largest HDF populations, only two countries have considerable numbers of patients on conventional HDF (Italy and Greece). As a result, the predominant HDF treatment mode within EMEA is on-line HDF with a share of around 95% of all HDF patients being treated with on-line HDF.

Observing the development of HDF patient numbers on a global scale between 2004 and 2010, the number of HDF patients increased by around 13% on average per year (table 4). While between 2004 and 2007 the average growth was only around 11% per year, there was a reported growth of around 15% on average per year between 2007 and 2010. All in all, the number of HDF patients grew about twice as fast as the number of HD patients over the last years.

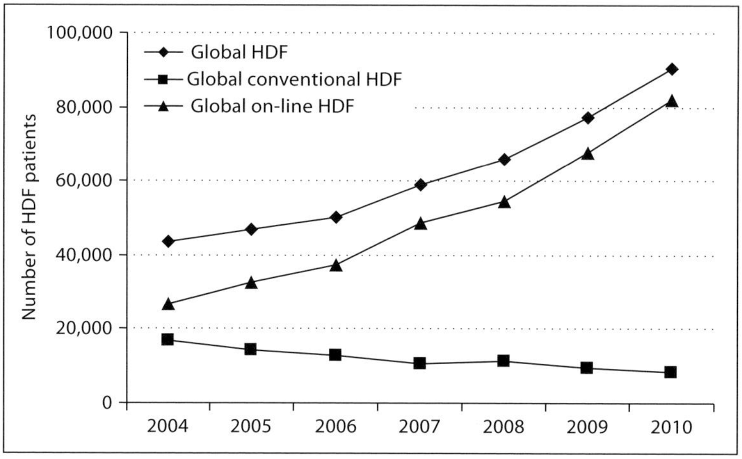

Fig. 1. Development of HDF patients from 2004 to 2010.

In EMEA and AP, the growth of the number of HDF patients between 2007 and 2010 was considerably higher than the corresponding growth between 2004 and 2007. While the HDF patient growth in AP between 2004 and 2007 was still below the HD patient growth on standard HD, in the region EMEA the HDF patient growth significantly exceeded the standard HD patient growth already at that time.

In EMEA, the number of patients treated by HDF (59,000 patients in 2010) is significantly higher than the number of patients treated by peritoneal dialysis (43,000 patients in 2010).

The two HDF modalities (i.e. conventional and on-line) display opposite trends. While on-line HDF patient numbers have increased strongly over the last 7 years at a rate of around 20% per annum, the number of patients treated with conventional HDF has decreased by around 11% per year. On-line HDF patient numbers increased in this period from around 27,000 patients to around 82,000. In the meantime, the number of patients treated with conventional HDF dropped from almost 17,000 patients in 2004 to around 8,500 in 2010 (fig. 1).

Conclusion

Use of HDF has increased consistently over the last years. In the majority of the countries analyzed, access to HDF therapy is still restricted due to various regulatory issues. Nevertheless, the percentage of chronic patients receiving HDF treatment grew by 13% per year on average between 2004 and 2010, which is about double the growth of the number of dialysis patients. In some regions and countries, more patients receive HDF nowadays than peritoneal dialysis and, in selected countries, HDF accounts for more than 25% of all extracorporeal dialysis treatments for ESRD patients. Besides the growing acceptance in the medical communities [8, 9], the positive development of this therapy option can also be seen as having been facilitated by the increasing availability of convenient technical solutions that support the administration of HDF in a resource-saving manner. In 2010, on-line HDF was by far the predominant mode of HDF therapy, being applied to around 90% of the global HDF patients.

Acknowledgements

We would like to express our thanks to national experts from more than 140 countries worldwide who have provided the data; without their collaboration, this report would not have been possible.

Disclosure Statement

Both authors are employees of Fresenius Medical Care.

References

1 US Renal Data System, USRDS 2009 Annual Data Report: Atlas of Chronic Kidney Disease and End-Stage Renal Disease in the United States, National Institutes of Health, National Institute of Diabetes and Digestive and Kidney Diseases (http://www.usrds.org/adr.htm).
2 European Renal Association – European Dialysis and Transplant Association Registry (http://www.era-edta-reg.org).
3 Australia & New Zealand Dialysis and Transplant Registry (http://www.anzdata.org.au).
4 DOPPS – Dialysis Outcomes and Practice Patterns Study (http://www.dopps.org).
5 Grassmann A, Gioberge S, Moeller S, Brown G: End-stage renal disease – global demographics in 2005 and observed trends. Artif Organs 2006;30:895–897.
6 Grassmann A, Gioberge S, Moeller S, Brown G: ESRD patients in 2004: global overview of patient numbers, treatment modalities and associated trends. Nephrol Dial Transplant 2005;20:2587–2593.
7 Moeller S, Gioberge S, Brown G: ESRD patients in 2001: global overview of patients, treatment modalities and development trends. Nephrol Dial Transplant 2002;17:2071–2076.
8 Canaud B, Bragg-Gresham JL, Marshall MR, et al: Mortality risk for patients receiving hemodiafiltration versus hemodialysis: European results from the DOPPS. Kidney Int 2006;69:2087–2093.
9 Jirka T, Cesare S, Di Benedetto A, et al: The impact of on-line haemodiafiltration on patient survival: results from a large network database. Nephrol Dial Transplant 2005;20(suppl 5):v18–v19.

Jan-Michael Sichart
Fresenius Medical Care Deutschland GmbH
Else-Kroener-Strasse 1
DE–61352 Bad Homburg (Germany)
Tel. + 49 6172 609 7817, E-Mail Jan-Michael Sichart@fmc-ag.com

Krick G, Ronco C (eds): On-Line Hemodiafiltration: The Journey and the Vision.
Contrib Nephrol. Basel, Karger, 2011, vol 175, pp 170–185

Seeking an Optimal Renal Replacement Therapy for the Chronic Kidney Disease Epidemic: The Case for On-Line Hemodiafiltration

Emanuele Gatti[a,b] · Claudio Ronco[c]

[a]Centre for Biomedical Technology at the Danube University of Krems, Krems, Austria;
[b]Fresenius Medical Care, Bad Homburg v.d.H., Germany; [c]Department of Nephrology Dialysis and Transplantation and International Renal Research Institute, San Bortolo Hospital, Vicenza, Italy

Abstract

The prevalence of chronic kidney disease (CKD) can be expected to increase dramatically in the foreseeable future, with suggestions that it has already reached epidemic proportions. The inadequate supply of donor organs, aggravated by an aging patient population, necessitates provision of sustainable dialysis treatment modalities. These treatment modalities must not only be of established clinical efficacy and effectiveness, but must simultaneously circumvent any potential treatment disparities due to geographical, social or other concurring factors. Home therapies might represent a partial solution to the complex issue of seeking optimal strategies to cope with the CKD epidemic. However, self-care renal replacement therapy (RRT), such as peritoneal dialysis (PD) and home therapies, can only be applied to a limited portion of the CKD population. Consequently, in preparation for coping with this CKD epidemic, specific large-scale plans need to be made that involve optimization of treatments already in use for the majority of the population requiring RRT, e.g. hemodialysis (HD). Extracorporeal chronic HD relies heavily on technology for its clinical success. Like the choice of the treatment modality and the complete medical approach to CKD patient care, the particular selection of the various components of the extracorporeal circuit has a significant impact on the well-being and survival of the patients. We present a medical-technological assessment of how best to treat vast numbers of dialysis patients under the financial restraints that are predicted to become even more severe as CKD entrenches itself as a more 'permanent epidemic'. A treatment modality is proposed that optimally addresses – and resolves – the debilitating effects of uremia, as well as of key clinical conditions closely linked to it. This treatment modality successfully tackles the issues of patient well-being, efficacy, effectiveness, safety and patient-nursing staff convenience – all in relation to the overall costs incurred by payers of renal care. In short, optimal care needs to be provided with shrinking resources and without compromising the medical appropriateness of the therapy. Additionally, we believe ensuring improved quality of life is just as important as prolonging patient survival. Therefore, a balanced compromise between optimal and affordable technology is required in order to reach the targets of achieving good medical care and meeting the expectations of patients, their families, healthcare providers, and society as a whole. Under these premises, and focusing on the aforementioned targets, we believe that on-line hemodiafiltration (HDF) represents the most advanced and clinically appropriate RRT modality available to best cope with the CKD epidemic. Together with the guidance and recommendations of those taking care of CKD patients on dialysis therapy, the contribution of industry is indispensable for the availability of highly reliable and affordable solutions to the impending dilemma. As representatives of the academic-medical community and of industry, we present a joint case for the application of on-line HDF towards meeting the challenge of large-scale provision of dialysis under an increasingly restrictive financial climate.

Adequate substitution of lost capabilities of diseased kidneys remains the fundamental objective of dialysis therapy. However, both peritoneal dialysis (PD) and hemodialysis (HD) are intrinsically imperfect as they cannot match the complex functions of the healthy kidney. Furthermore, besides blood purification and fluid control, several accompanying issues need to be addressed or resolved. Today, with the chronic kidney disease (CKD) 'epidemic' becoming more widespread and involving an aging population, the core necessity – and challenge – is how best to deliver a more intensive renal replacement therapy (RRT) under increasing economical restraints imposed by stretched healthcare budgets worldwide [1, 2]. Optimal RRT must therefore be the result of a compromise between the needs of all involved in the care of CKD patients requiring dialysis. Many unmet clinical needs should be addressed together with the best utilization of available technology and financial budgets [3]. The involvement and participation of patients as well as their families is crucial if home therapies could represent a possible solution to the complex problem. However, self-care RRT, such as PD and home-based therapies, only apply to a limited portion of the dialysis population. For the remaining majority, optimization of in-center HD should be attempted, considering clinical as well as ethical and financial issues.

Hemodiafiltration (HDF) is a treatment modality applied to 14% of CKD patients on regular RRT in Europe in 2010 and, as such, significantly more patients received HDF than PD in this region [4]. The principles and clinical characterization of HDF have been known for over four decades [5]. Since then, online HDF has been validated as the most efficient extracorporeal modality for the removal of both small and large uremic retention solutes ('uremic toxins'). Today, a growing body of scientific evidence and clinical experience provides

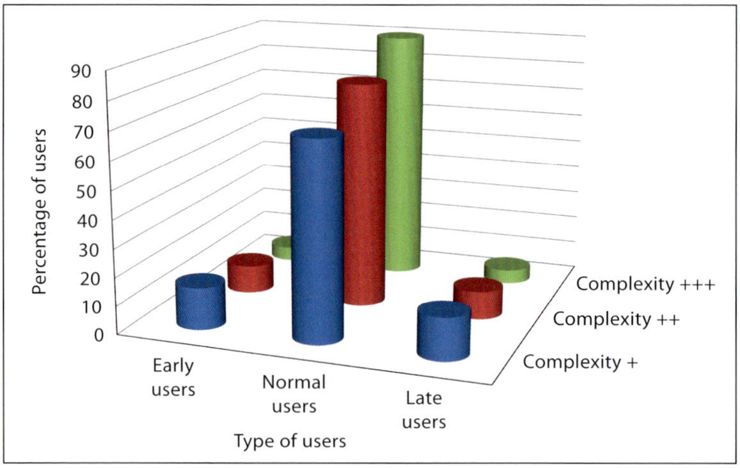

Fig. 1. Gaussian distribution of technology users based on technology complexity. Early users are mostly stimulated by curiosity, desire of progress and willingness to try new approaches. Mass users are generally following the clear evidence of a benefit for a given technology. Late users are generally resistant to changes even in the presence of good evidence for a benefit offered by a technology. In some cases this resistance implicates other factors including insecurity, specific resistance to something new, or even extra medical factors including business or conflict of interest.

a better understanding of this treatment modality, and a host of clinical benefits have been documented [6]. Moreover, constant technical refinements have made on-line HDF safe and easy to perform in routine clinical practice [5]. Nevertheless, an even wider application of the technique is precluded by the defense of more traditional techniques and the perpetual demand for more conclusive survival data from large-scale, prospective, randomized, controlled trials (RCTs) [7, 8]. This, however, is a typical evolution in the utilization of most new technologies where there is a well-distributed gaussian curve, as depicted in figure 1.

In the presence of an overwhelming body of clinical experience and data in favor of on-line HDF, including indications of a survival benefit (albeit the level of evidence is deemed not to be sufficient to satisfy the criteria of the purist) how, then, could on-line HDF be expected to evolve? We believe that the extended clinical experience, scientific validation and technological maturity of on-line HDF offers the best opportunity to satisfy the collective interests of the patient, the family, all healthcare providers and of society as a whole [9]. As representatives of the academic, medical and industry communities, we consider a joint case for the application of on-line HDF towards meeting the challenge of large-scale provision of dialysis under an increasingly restrictive financial climate [2].

Renal Replacement Therapy in the New Millennium: Unmet Clinical Needs

All the prognoses regarding dialysis patient growth made over the last two decades proved to be inaccurate and underestimated the magnitude of the CKD epidemic. Despite significant prolongation of life of CKD patients due to dialysis, major medical issues regarding adequacy and effectiveness are still open with many clinical problems still unresolved [2]. The endless cyclicity of dialysis therapy and its intermittent nature compared to the continuous functioning of the natural kidney causes permanent alterations in the hemodynamic and cardiovascular functions of the patient. This, together with the accumulation of uremic toxins of various molecular weight ranges and the impairment of the hormonal and regulatory functions of the native organ, may lead to long-term complications, especially causing skeletal, metabolic and cardiovascular disorders [10]. These and other unmet clinical needs are the cause of treatment inadequacy and unsatisfactory long-term outcomes. Even when life is prolonged for several years, the overall health status of the patient may be impaired considerably with insufficient quality of life (QoL).

Renal Replacement Therapy in the New Millennium: Social, Ethical and Financial Issues

In spite of enormous efforts targeting the optimization of technology and directed towards the individualization of treatments and treatment schedules, many patients in the world still do not have access to basic RRT facilities. Even when RRT is provided, discrimination due to age or geographic origins may occur. These problems are exacerbated in modern society by lifestyle conditions and financial constraints that make healthcare providers unable to cope with the discrepancy between expectations and resources. Today all these issues are further complicated by a worldwide economic crisis, growing patient numbers and inadequate healthcare planning. In these circumstances, both industry and clinical medicine are confronted with moral and ethical issues and are expected to offer suitable solutions. In chronic dialysis, we propose on-line HDF as a reliable technique capable of meeting the main current clinical and financial challenges as well as the diverse expectations of multiple stakeholders (patients, physicians, industry, healthcare providers and funders). Another important issue is the relative distribution of available resources between dialysis technology and the pharmacological requirements of dialysis patients. It seems that, with the allocation of fixed budgets for the entire therapy, an optimal combination of these two components must be achieved, i.e. solutions must look for an integration of both components rather than a competitive substitution.

On-Line HDF: Short- and Long-Term Clinical Benefits

It is important to reiterate the case for on-line HDF, which has established itself as a consolidated therapy over the last two decades [5–7]. The main benefits attributed to on-line HDF include efficient elimination of larger uremic toxins, anemia correction with an associated reduced requirement for erythropoiesis-stimulating agents, lower calcium-phosphate product levels, increased hemodynamic stability and better blood pressure control [8, 9]. A reduced incidence of side effects and an improvement of nutritional status have also been documented [11]. The reduced activation of inflammation and oxidative stress pathways with convective therapies, linked mainly to a reduced uremic toxin load, has been postulated to have a protective effect on both the vasculature and endothelium. Collectively, these mechanisms seem to contribute to a reduction in the frequency and severity of the cardiovascular complications that affect the majority of dialysis patients. Finally, there is considerable evidence indicating an improved QoL for patients on on-line HDF compared to conventional therapies.

On-Line HDF: Evidence of Survival Benefits

A number of investigations have reported reduced mortality rates amongst patients treated with on-line HDF. A review of all the current trials on high-flux HD and HDF has recently been published [7]. An observational study by Canaud et al. [12] involving over 2,000 patients indicated a 35% improved survival with high-volume on-line HDF independently of its higher dialysis dose. Prospectively collected data from 56 clinics in four European countries (EuCliD database) confirmed these results in terms of potential survival benefits with on-line HDF [13]. Two other RCTs (the Turkish HDF vs. high-fux-HD study and the Dutch CONTRAST study with HDF vs. low-flux HD) examining the impact of on-line HDF on patient survival have just been completed [14, 15]. Preliminary results did not show a significant difference in survival rates as a whole between HDF-treated patients and those treated with either high-flux HD or low-flux HD. However, in both studies, the volume of substitution delivered (17–20 liters per session) during the entire HDF session was identified as an independent risk factor, confirming earlier findings of the DOPPS study [12]. The volume of substitution, a surrogate of the convective dialysis dose, should thus be considered as a critical factor that may impact patient mortality rates. While acknowledging that these results only indicate an association between survival and therapy modality, and that selected patients may have received the largest amount of substitution fluids because of better cardiovascular stability and a better vascular access, one has to recognize that three independent, large-scale studies have now indicated that high-volume on-line HDF may represent a survival advantage.

On-Line HDF: A Therapy Meeting Multiple Requirements

On-Line HDF Fulfils the Quest for More Intensive Dialysis

The need for more intensive dialysis is widely recognized. Efficient detoxification of blood, i.e. removal of relevant uremic retention solutes, remains the fundamental objective of all HD therapies. Uremic toxicity is better understood today, yet there are still no clear indications as to specifically which substances need to be removed during HD [16]. With individual substances often controversially acquiring overt attention in terms of their potential in vivo toxicity and clinical relevance [17], the only certainty is that, irrespective of their number or identity, small *and* large accumulated substances need to be removed as efficiently as possible during HD therapies. As the majority (56%) of all HD patients worldwide are treated with high-flux HD (which also entails a convective component for solute removal, albeit smaller than in HDF), a more efficient removal of larger uremic toxins is considered beneficial. It has to be noted that the concept of urea Kt/V, commonly used to assess the delivered dose and efficiency of HD treatment, does not represent efficiency of elimination of larger uremic toxins that contribute to the uremic syndrome. Another general approach to delivering more intensive dialysis is to increase duration and frequency of treatment, both of which are associated with better outcomes [18]. Although not verified conclusively by prospective RCTs, more intensive HD regimens, including daily short or prolonged nocturnal (in-center or home) HD, are perceived as being advantageous in terms of both reduced morbidity and mortality. This, again, would only be applicable to a very limited group of patients and in areas where the required resources (including qualified personnel) are available. Given the theoretical and practical advantages of long or more frequent schedules and while accepting the possibility of these treatments fulfilling some of the unmet clinical needs, we do not anticipate that this represents a solution for the vast majority of the CKD population.

On-line HDF is the most intensive form of HD treatment available by virtue of its ability to more thoroughly remove a broad spectrum of substances involved in uremia. Convective (unlike diffusive) transport across appropriate high-flux membranes facilitates removal of larger uremic solutes; together with higher ultrafiltration rates – and thus increased convection made possible by usage of larger volumes of replacement fluid in on-line HDF – more efficient blood cleansing is achieved. The finding in three survival studies that a survival advantage is evident only at high-volume on-line HDF is thus consistent with these mechanistic considerations [12, 14, 15]. The degree of convective transport is thus decisive from an overall clinical point of view. Prolonged (e.g. nocturnal)

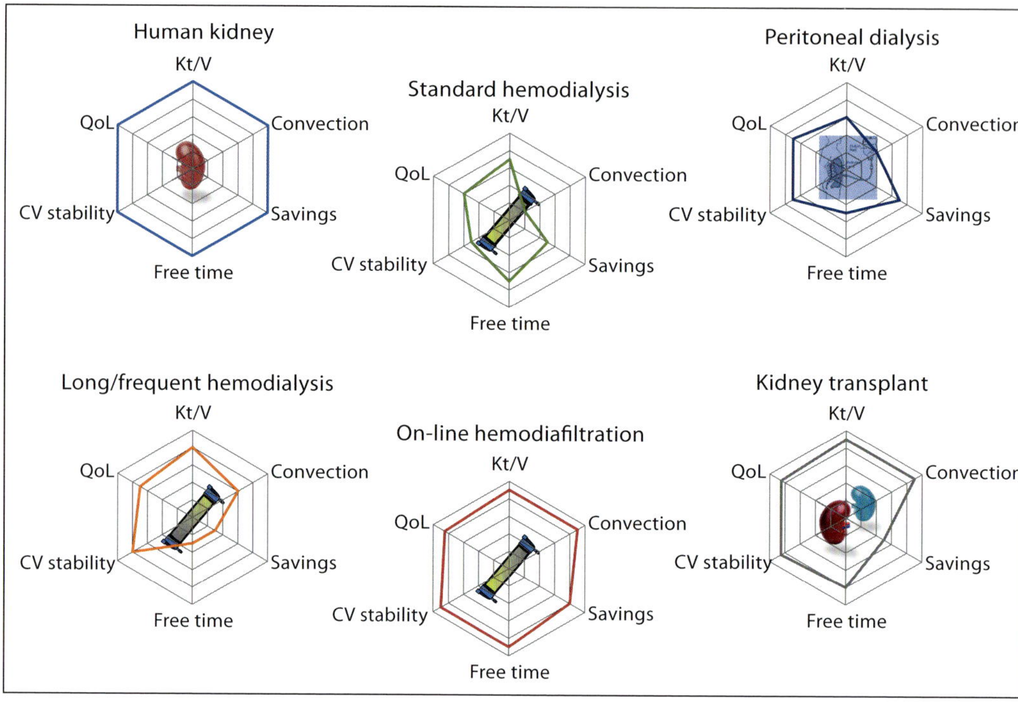

Fig. 2. Radar graph describing the performances of six different conditions: normal kidney, standard HD, PD, long/frequent HD, on-line HDF, and kidney transplant. Given a full score for the normal kidney function, we can see that on-line HDF is the therapy replacing the native organ in the most efficient way after kidney transplant. Kidney transplant, PD and long/frequent HD are performing well but their applicability is limited. Savings for all therapies includes healthcare costs, hospitalization, comorbidities and use of EPO and other expensive drugs. QoL includes survival and rehabilitation.

dialysis in the form of either high-flux HD or on-line HDF would only partially enhance detoxification processes for larger solutes by overcoming the limitations of transport of intracellular toxins into the blood compartment. This, however, would be at the expense of increased time spent on dialysis, an unacceptable social life and higher costs for the society. Thus, even assuming that a small set of patients could benefit from long or daily dialysis, on-line HDF appears to incorporate most of the advantages of long and slow treatments while taking only a few hours of patient's time and keeping the costs under control. Again, a complex compromise is the result of optimization of different performances of a therapy (fig. 2). In figure 2, radar plots of different treatments modalities are presented, comparing performance indices with the performance of the human kidney. Not only are the results with on-line HDF superior to those with other treatments in specific aspects, but on-line HDF as a whole shows a more homogeneous distribution of the different performance indices.

On-Line HDF Combines the Need for Efficient Detoxification with Reduced Inflammation

CKD is a pro-inflammatory condition; underlying inflammation corresponds with progression of renal failure [19]. Several conditions related to CKD (including malnutrition, anemia, mineral bone disease and vascular access) correlate with imbalances of various immune regulatory pathways leading to accelerated vascular disease and atherosclerosis. As cardiovascular disease and complications are the major cause of mortality in dialysis patients, curtailing underlying inflammation and associated oxidative stress is emerging as a strategy to improve patient outcomes.

To derive the full benefits of convective therapies in terms of achieving more intensive dialysis, large volumes of substitution/replacement fluids are mandatory and, as mentioned above, have been linked to improved patient survival. Exposure of patients to such large volumes of fluids poses a potential risk of increased inflammation should the dialysis fluids be contaminated with bacterial endotoxins [20]. To avoid this, an essential prerequisite of modern convective therapies is the availability for large quantities of inexpensive and highly pure (microbiologically) substitution fluids. Ultrafilters with high endotoxin retention capacities allow the 'online' production of replacement solutions from dialysate that meet such safety and quality requirements. This has been the key factor towards reviving and facilitating convective therapies. Since most dialysis centers today already use ultrapure dialysis fluids, the transition to on-line HDF is more feasible and a growing number of HD patients could benefit from the clinical advantages of this treatment modality [21].

On-Line HDF Offers Patients a Better QoL

In addition to improved survival, patients on on-line HDF experience fewer side effects, feel more energetic, have a better appetite (and are consequently better nourished and require less erythropoietin (EPO)) and sleep better at night [8, 11]. All these secondary aspects result in a significant improvement in the QoL as perceived by the patient. Again, other therapies (such as PD or long/frequent HD schedules) may offer similar results. However, as demonstrated in figure 2, the performances of these therapies in terms of improvement of QoL are achieved at the expense of increased costs or increased time spent on dialysis. These two factors represent a burden for society as well as for the patient and the family, not to mention that such treatments are only applicable to a minority of patients. However, it is also true that some typical weak points of short intermittent on-line HDF sessions (in which high rates of fluid removal are still required) are indeed partially overcome by these treatments: the associated improvements in hemodynamic stability and the decreased sense of thirst at the end of the session result in a well-tolerated treatment and a lower incidence of interdialytic uncontrolled fluid gain.

On-Line HDF Has the Potential to Allow Curtailment of Long-Term Costs of HD Therapy

Healthcare systems all over the world face considerable challenges resulting from the current demographic and economic developments [1, 2]. The growing prevalence of chronically ill patients, including CKD and particularly those needing RRT, is increasingly considered as a critical public health problem: in the last decade the prevalence of end-stage renal disease (ESRD) in Europe grew at an annual average rate of 5.3% and, at the end of 2010, the number of patients treated for ESRD was estimated to be 642,000 in Europe. Of these patients, approximately 426,000 (around 66% of all ESRD patients) receive RRT [4].

Despite the rising burden of illness and the growing total cost of RRT, the quest for sustainable strategies of care for this patient population has still not satisfactorily been addressed and a comprehensive understanding of the economics of CKD is still unavailable. This is due to lack of an integrated approach to CKD as a chronic illness and a missing balance between clinical and economic goals. Optimization of RRT in the presence of constrained resources nevertheless requires coupling of highest possible medical standards with highest efficiency and ethical distribution of resources. Still today, the costs of different therapeutic interventions at different stages of CKD have not been comprehensively addressed. On the contrary, the tendency can be observed in numerous publications to focus exclusively on costs related to a single dialysis treatment or medication, ignoring the perspective of long-term costs, social costs and overall outcomes. This problem, while understandable in the context of a fee-for-service refunding frame, underestimates the complexity of CKD as a chronic illness that impedes an understanding of the true nature of costs of care for patients with CKD. Furthermore, the ongoing confrontation of the seemingly irreconcilable perspectives of growing total cost of RRT and the need for high quality standards often hinders openness for the optimization potentials that result from the skillful orchestration of the various aspects of care. Optimization efforts in renal care have different dimensions: both the intertemporal cost interdependencies as well as the interdependencies of cost in different care settings (especially ambulatory versus inpatient cost-of-care) need to be considered. In addition, in the simultaneous pursuit of the objectives of sustainable quality and total care efficiency, the consequences of therapeutic decisions and choice of technological solutions during every single treatment have to be addressed. In the case of on-line HDF, the simultaneous short- and long-term effects of treatment must be evaluated looking at overall outcomes, safety, convenience as well as direct and indirect expenditure and benefits for the society. It is pertinent to note here that a number of studies have indicated that on-line HDF allows correction of anemia at reduced EPO doses, with the results of the recent trial of Ok et al. [14] showing a 20% reduction in EPO requirements while maintaining the target hemoglobin and hematocrit levels [8].

Wider Use of On-Line HDF Offers Refinements in Device Costs

As is true with the introduction of all advanced medical technologies, there is a degree of apprehension regarding higher costs incurred by the technical components of on-line HDF. Bearing in mind the aforementioned clinical and financial benefits to society as a whole, on-line HDF still offers potential refinements of future cost developments as penetration levels increase over the course of time. With the rapid increase of on-line HDF over the last decade, we have already observed that, as demand increases, an accompanying lowering of production costs (and prices) has been realized. This is the result of increased economies of scale, lower amortization of investments, automatization, optimization of component designs, delocalization of production and leaner production processes. This trend will continue and expand in the future: the dialysis field has encountered such trends in the past, for example with bicarbonate dialysis fluids, the demand for which led to cost reductions over time.

Potential Future Technical Refinements of On-Line HDF

Dialysis relies heavily on diverse technologies for the delivery of an adequate short- and long-term therapy. Indeed, the choice and quality of the individual components may have a significant impact on long-term outcomes. While the effects and limitations of long-term HD are recognized, we are unaware of the potential benefits of a long-term application of on-line HDF. In this circumstance, we must offer new chances to our patients. Ever since recognition of the advantages of convective transport and the birth of hemofiltration and then HDF, the technique has periodically undergone technical refinements in response to clinical needs. A significant number of therapy variations have evolved around classical HDF and on-line HDF [5, 21]. This trend will continue and further advances can be expected in the future.

On-line HDF can further be streamlined to avoid unnecessary alarms, interruptions, disruptions or discomfort during the course of treatment, and to avoid inefficient and non-effective use of resources. Intelligent technologies available today enable more precise monitoring of treatment parameters and provide the foundation for future innovations aimed at maximizing quality, dose and safety of treatment. An understanding of the following is essential to achieve such refinements:

(A) The intricate interdependencies between all components, from vascular access preparation and care, to the often 'trivial' issue of choice of needle, to how the artificial kidney and the dialysis system can work in perfect harmony.

(B) The dialyzer-machine interface and interplay between these two systems as linked by IT systems that can establish trends and the right selection of treatment parameters in response to clinical and technical signals (from treatment individualization, to profiling, to biofeedback).

Essentially, four areas of technical refinement can be identified that address unmet clinical needs, the solution of which would elevate on-line HDF to the next level of efficiency and efficacy.

Fluid Removal – How Much and How Fast?

A more effective fluid management is crucial to patient outcomes as non-physiological fluid shifts promote hemodynamic instability, development of vascular stiffness and left ventricular hypertrophy. To achieve volume control by ultrafiltration (i.e. primarily the magnitude of convective transport) in on-line HDF, the first objective is to ascertain, as precisely as possible, the overall and the net amount of fluid to be removed/replaced. The second is to ensure that the desired fluid exchange (according to patient requirements) is fully achieved in each treatment session. Online monitoring of blood parameters will allow adjustment of UFR to identify the patient-specific exchange rate possible at any given point in time in the presence of clinical stability. Determining instantaneously achievable exchange rates will therefore permit a better response to the highest achievable conditions of efficiency. The use of bioimpedance technology permits accurate, non-invasive and objective assessment of fluid status, defining the amount of fluid to be removed [22]. Furthermore, it enables a link between the fluid status and blood pressure, thereby allowing a more rational prescription of antihypertensive medication. Coupling bioimpedance with continuous and non-invasive blood volume monitoring allows not only to target overall fluid removal but also enables control of fluid removal rate. However, filter properties and other treatment parameters also need to be taken into consideration to prescribe and deliver optimal therapy. Derived measures such as filtration fraction, intravascular refilling rate and local protein concentration may all contribute to achieve the best filter performance and to design proportionally adequate filtration and reinfusion strategies.

Maximum Blood Flow Available for Solute and Water Removal

Both the total amount of fluid to be removed (allowing for weight gain between sessions) and the subsequent substitution of replacement fluid during an on-line HDF session depend upon adequate 'delivery' of blood flow from the patient into the extracorporeal circuit. An understanding of diverse vascular access-related issues is a prerequisite to attain the maximal blood flow rate through the dialyzer: the extent of solute clearance achieved is to a considerable extent determined by high effective blood flow rates (Q_b). As the fistula needles or catheters used are normally the limiting factors for the extracorporeal blood flow rates, their dimensions (inner diameter, length) are key to achievable diffusive and convective solute clearances. Advanced monitoring systems allowing the optimal regulation of blood and dialysate flows will contribute to treatment optimization. Blood flow rate can thus be automatically adapted to assure control of arterial pressure and to assure the best available blood flow delivered to the dialyzer. Of course, recirculation is an important measure in complete management of dialysis parameters and in avoiding mistakes in effective treatment delivery.

Automatic Dialysate/Substitution Fluid Flow Rate Management
Both dialysate and substitution fluid flow rates (Q_d and Q_s) are optimized and individualized based on clinical criteria of how much fluid needs to be – and can be – removed/reinfused during each session. In combination with the aforementioned management of hydration status, the reinfusion rate should be adjusted to blood flow rate (thereby controlling hemoconcentration) while blood flow rate is adjusted to dialysis fluid flow rate (thereby controlling diffusive efficiency). Essentially, the task is to identify *maximum achievable exchange volume* based on patient blood parameters evaluated by online monitoring via pressure and resistance in the circuit. When pressure increases, then the machine responds by adapting Q_b (reducing) and altering Q_d and Q_s, and/or creating pulses across the dialyzer. The objective is to utilize to the maximal what the patient can offer and what the dialyzer can provide without wastage of the potential of either. As such a treatment strategy approach could impact cardiovascular disorders, drug dosing (e.g. antihypertensive medication) and be a component of strategies supporting efficient administration of EPO.

Maximization/Optimization of Available Filter Performance
It has been recognized for some time now that the potential of the dialyzer, the focal point of the blood-cleansing function of all HD therapies, has yet to be fully harnessed. Dialyzer design studies are under way to optimize dialyzer surfaces and geometries which will enable best performance based on patient parameters. New approaches are also being investigated to select optimum dialyzer properties to suit specific treatment and patient parameters, thereby optimizing interplay of all relevant parameters of the dialysis procedure. In addition, new design of dialyzer surfaces and geometries will enable best performances based on patient parameters.

Filter performance decreases over the duration of each treatment, being at its highest during the early phases of the dialysis session. This is attributed to the formation of a 'secondary membrane' comprising several adsorbed proteins as well as other blood components; its composition is determined not only by the membrane polymer and structure, but is also influenced by rheological factors including blood viscosity and fiber-filter geometry. Thus, hollow-fiber dimensions (wall thickness and lumen diameter) and filter geometry must be designed or selected to reduce longitudinal and TMP increases during treatment. Again, treatment parameters must be selected to optimize the performance of the filter; pressure monitoring sensors within the machine can identify filter properties at beginning of treatment (i.e. calibrate the filter at t = 0) and undertake measures to maintain the dialyzer performance as close as possible to this initial (optimal) performance throughout the entire treatment (i.e. maximum and consistent performance of the dialyzer). Pressure bursts would pulsate the membrane at appropriate time points, disturbing formation of secondary membrane and thus maintaining the membrane surface in a defined, consistent state. In situations where there is a tendency for blood coagulation to occur (e.g. at suboptimal heparinization regimens), pressure pulses across the membrane would further serve to unclog any clots that may have developed. Avenues are also being explored to reduce the tendency for clot formation by pulsing buffered citrate-containing dialysis fluid across the membrane to achieve a local surface anticoagulant effect that would lead to reduced need or even an absence for anticoagulant. These cross-filtration pulses might be coupled with predetermined (frequency, direction and amplitude) shock waves to further obtain disruption of laminar flow and fluid stagnation in the dialyzer [23, 24].

Thus, the vision is to refine on-line HDF as a system which is continuously self-regulating based on intelligent adaption of parameters evaluated by blood and dialysis fluid online monitoring. Realization of such targets would represent the next most important refinement of HDF therapy, following the landmark of making unlimited amounts of inexpensive and microbiologically pure substitution fluids available 'online' that facilitated application of convective transport.

Conclusions: Adding Quality to Extended Life

With the expected worldwide escalation of CKD, provision of dialysis therapy on a large-scale requires due consideration. Preemptive strategies need to be put into place regarding delivery of the most optimal form of therapy to cope with a chronic disease necessitating regular, high technology-dependent interventions for the entire lifetime of a patient to ensure survival. Clinical as well as economical factors are inseparable deliberations for the provision of dialysis therapy of the future. In essence a stable therapy, that is by no means substandard, is required for the bulk of the dialysis population. Such a treatment modality must have demonstrable clinical effectiveness, efficacy and safety. Furthermore, it must be individualized, be convenient for patients and nursing staff alike, and be affordable – not necessarily in that order. A state of preparedness (incorporating these factors and based on the dialysis experience to date) is required to cater for the projected increase of a dialysis population having more elderly people with multiple comorbid conditions.

Foremost, it is essential to recognize the specific needs of the today's dialysis patient. As with any chronic disease, dialysis patients wish to live full, normal lives with minimal restriction to their lifestyle, particularly in terms of family life, leisure and employment. Dialysis therapy, by its very nature, does not always permit this. In-center dialysis, or even home treatment, disrupts daily routine – as does more prolonged, more frequent or nocturnal dialysis therapy.

Meeting the complex and specific clinical needs of the dialysis patient today involves several components, each of which requires due consideration. The technological features of the dialysis procedure, while being the core of the life-saving function of dialysis, are only one of several factors around delivery of HD therapy. The entire clinical picture of each individual patient and the type and quality of overall medical care provided, including therapies for CKD-associated comorbid conditions, collectively determine morbidity and mortality outcomes. Dialysis technology, or a particular treatment modality, is not the only determinant of patient outcomes or of survival.

Prolonging survival for any disease with a particular therapeutic option has, alone, little meaning without ensuring that the patient derives an adequate QoL. Patients might prefer a higher QoL for the duration of the period they are on dialysis, rather than simply living longer but being bedridden and unable to lead active lifestyles. Dialysis patients themselves, once on on-line HDF, do not wish to revert to other less advanced modalities; increased patient well-being, with fewer complications, has been documented with on-line HDF.

Thus, prescription of a particular treatment modality should not be based on the sole criteria of whether evidence is available from large-scale prospective RCTs, showing that the modality is able to prolong life. The fastidious quest, in certain quarters, for more conclusive data indicating that on-line HDF prolongs patient survival may result in a missed opportunity to give patients a therapy that has demonstrable clinical advantages in several ways (as outlined in this communication). Clinical experience is indispensable; an extensive clinical application spanning over two decades has shown that on-line HDF therapy has been successfully prescribed for thousands of patients.

Evidence indicating reduced mortality is not mandatory for the allocation of a particular treatment option. Clinical efficacy and effectiveness, both well established for on-line HDF, are more pertinent. Nevertheless, it has to be noted that there *are* indications that on-line HDF reduces mortality rates under certain conditions – only that the evidence is deemed not to be sufficiently strong. Once the clinical viability of a therapy has been established, allocators of renal care consider the costs of delivery of the therapeutic intervention. As the true overall costs of delivery of dialysis therapy are extremely complex to calculate and are as yet unavailable, technological components, consumables or medication are usually the most obvious subject of cost-containing measures. Estimation of the potential cost-saving attributed to patient well-being is difficult to ascertain and is unfortunately not available. For instance, rehabilitation due to better general health and being more active enables patients to attain a degree of normality in their lifestyle and make contributions back to society. Ability to return to, or maintain, employment overcomes manpower shortages in certain sectors, provides income from tax contributions and makes dialysis patients less dependent on state contributions. Better general health, in short, reduces the burden to society and healthcare providers.

We are faced with the challenge of delivering an optimal therapy that meets the interests of the patient, medical personnel, as well as the care providers. Medical appropriateness has essentially to be balanced with economic sustainability for the care providers, payers and society as a whole. Under these premises, more frequent dialysis, e.g. in the form of daily dialysis, may clinically be in the interests of the patient but immediately raises (serious) issues regarding increased costs, logistics of delivery of therapy and availability of medical personnel. HD therapy is, and has always been, a balance between what should, and can, be delivered to the patient. On-line HDF may not fulfill all the criteria of an ideal treatment modality, but with the current knowledge of what dialysis can and should deliver and under the present pressures of cost containment, it is the most optimal modality in the interests of all the stakeholders involved in renal care. On-line HDF, based on sound principles and clinical experience documented in clinical databases, affords significant advantages to the patient – including QoL and possibly extended longevity. Significantly, future technological advances outlined in this article will make this therapy option even more efficient and reliable regarding improving the QoL of the dialysis patient. Since its revival, on-line HDF has followed the path of steady incremental advances and of resolving technical issues to facilitate the clinical implementation of the modality. This trend may be challenged by future developments involving recently announced leading-edge technologies, like regenerative medicine, adsorption or portable dialysis devices. These quantum leaps, if realized into reliable products, may elevate blood purification in CKD to a better and more individualized cleansing modality. However, most likely a combination of new and established best practices, such as on-line HDF, will represent the optimum approach for treating the vast patient numbers of the CKD epidemic.

Acknowledgement

The authors are sincerely grateful to Sudhir Bowry for his dedicated assistance in developing the manuscript and its final preparation.

References

1 St Peter WL: Introduction: chronic kidney disease: a burgeoning health epidemic. J Manag Care Pharm 2007:13:S2–S5.
2 Levey AS, Coresh J: Chronic kidney disease. Lancet 2011 (E-pub ahead of print).
3 Ritz E, Zeier M: Unmet clinical needs in dialysis: what can we do? Contrib Nephrol. Basel, Karger, 2001, vol 133, pp 1–9.
4 Fresenius Medical Care Research: Market & Competitor Survey, unpubl. data, 2010.
5 Ronco C, Cruz D: Hemodiafiltration history, technology and clinical results. Adv Chronic Kidney Dis 2007;14:231–243.
6 Blankestijn PJ, Ledebo I, Canaud B: Hemodiafiltration: clinical evidence and remaining questions. Kidney Int 2010;77:581–587.

7 Locatelli F, Manzoni C, Del Vecchio L, Cavalli A, Pontoriero G: Recent trials on hemodiafiltration. Contrib Nephrol. Basel, Karger, 2011, vol 171, pp 92–100.
8 Bowry SK, Gatti E: Impact of hemodialysis therapy on anemia of chronic kidney disease: the potential mechanisms. Blood Purif 2011;32:210–219.
9 Canaud B, Chenine L, Henriet D, Leray H: Online hemodiafiltration: a multipurpose therapy for improving quality of renal replacement therapy. Contrib Nephrol. Basel, Karger, 2008, vol 161, pp 191–198.
10 Wali RK, Henrich WL: Chronic kidney disease: a risk factor for cardiovascular disease. Cardiol Clin 2005;23:343–362.
11 Tiranathanagul K, Praditpornsilpa K, Katavetin P, Srisawat N, Townamchai N, Susantitaphong P, Tungsanga K, Eiam-Ong S: Online hemodiafiltration in Southeast Asia: a three-year prospective study of a single center. Ther Apher Dial 2009;13:56–62.
12 Canaud B, Bragg-Gresham JL, Marshall MR, Desmeules S, Gillespie BW, Depner T, Klassen P, Port FK: Mortality risk for patients receiving hemodiafiltration versus hemodialysis: European results from the DOPPS. Kidney Int 2006;69:2087–2093.
13 Jirka T, Cesare S, Di Benedetto A, et al: Mortality risk for patients receiving hemodiafiltration versus hemodialysis: European results from the DOPPS. Kidney Int 2006;70:1524.
14 Ok E, Asci G, Sevinc-Ok E, Kircelli F, Yilmaz M, Hur E, Sezis M, Demirci M, Ozdogan O, Demirci C, Onen Sertoz O, Duman S, Ozkahya M, Kayikcioglu M, Elbi H, Basci A, Toz H: Comparison of postdilution online hemodiafiltration and hemodialysis (Turkish HDF Study). ERA-EDTA 2011, LBCT2.
15 Grooteman M, Van den Dorpel R, Bots M, Penne L, Van der Weerd N, Mazairac A, den Hoedt C, van der Tweel I, Lévesque R, Nubé M, Ter Wee P, Blankestijn P: Online hemodiafiltration versus low-flux hemodialysis: effects on all-cause mortality and cardiovascular events in a randomized controlled trial. The convective transport study (CONTRAST). ERA-EDTA 2011, LBCT1.
16 Vanholder R, van Laecke S, Glorieux G: What is new in uremic toxicity? Pediatr Nephrol 2008;23:1211–21.
17 Vanholder R, Bammens B, de Loor H, Glorieux G, Meijers B, Schepers E, Massy Z, Evenepoel P: Warning: the unfortunate end of *p*-cresol as a uraemic toxin. Nephrol Dial Transplant 2011;26:1464–1467.
18 Lacson E Jr, Brunelli SM: Hemodialysis treatment time: a fresh perspective. Clin J Am Soc Nephrol 2011 (E-pub ahead of print).
19 Stenvinkel P: New insights on inflammation in chronic kidney disease – genetic and nongenetic factors. Nephrol Ther 2006;2:111–119.
20 Schindler R. Inflammation and dialysate quality. Hemodial Int 2006;10:S56–S59.
21 Ledebo I, Blankestijn PJ: Haemodiafiltration – optimal efficiency and safety. NDT Plus 2010;3:8–16.
22 Wabel P, Chamney P, Moissl U, Jirka T: Importance of whole-body bioimpedance spectroscopy for the management of fluid balance. Blood Purif 2009;27:75–80.
23 Kim JC, Garzotto F, Ronco C: Dynamic hemodialysis: a potential solution for middle molecule removal. Contrib Nephrol. Basel, Karger, 2011, vol 171, pp 107–112.
24 Kim JC, Garzotto F, Cruz DN, Goh CY, Nalesso F, Kim JH, Kang E, Kim HC, Ronco C: Enhancement of solute removal in a hollow-fiber hemodialyzer by mechanical vibration. Blood Purif 2011;314:227–234.

Claudio Ronco, MD
Department of Nephrology Dialysis and Transplantation and
International Renal Research Institute (IRRIV), San Bortolo Hospital
Viale Rodolfi, 37, IT–36100 Vicenza (Italy)
Tel. +39 0 444 753869, E-Mail cronco@goldnet.it

Author Index

Subject Index